AYURV

The
Gentle Health
System

HANS H. RHYNER

MOTILAL BANARSIDASS PUBLISHERS PRIVATE LIMITED • DELHI

First Indian Edition: Delhi, 1998
Reprint: Delhi, 2003

ISBN: 81-208-1500-9 (Cloth)
ISBN: 81-208-1501-7 (Paper)

Also available at:
MOTILAL BANARSIDASS
41 U.A. Bungalow Road, Jawahar Nagar, Delhi 110 007
8 Mahalaxmi Chamber, 22 Bhulabhai Desai Road, Mumbai 400 026
236, 9th Main III Block, Jayanagar, Bangalore 560 011
120' Royapettah High Road, Mylapore, Chennai 600 004
Sanas Plaza, 1302 Baji Rao Road, Pune 411 002
8 Camac Street, Kolkata 700 017
Ashok Rajpath, Patna 800 004
Chowk, Varanasi 221 001

Published 1994 by Sterling Publising Company, Inc. U.S.A.
Originally published 1992
by BLV Berlagsgesellschaft mbH, München, Germany

Photos by Verena Eggmann, Hans H. Rhyner, and Lois Stadler

Printed in India
BY EXCEL PRINTERS PVT. LTD.
C-206 NARAINA, PHASE-I, NEW DELHI 110028
Ph.: 25795899, 9810082582, e-mail: excelprinters.biz

Contents

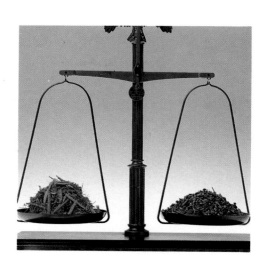

Introduction

The development of medicine as a social science occurred over many centuries. Every culture has influenced this development, particularly the evolution of the many different methods of healing. *Allopathic* medicine (today, synonymous with Western medicine) has its foundations in Greek culture. Hippocrates and Galen were scientists and physicians as well as philosophers. They considered philosophy and medicine two sides of the same coin. Anyone practising or teaching medicine also had to master philosophy, the latter playing an important role in the successful treatment of a patient.

Only in the last few centuries, with the emergence of natural sciences, such as physics, chemistry, and biology, has medicine been separated from philosophy. Modern medicine has become primarily a *somatological science,* resting on an experimental basis. Every healing method is subjected to clinical trials and rejected if proven ineffective. This leads to an exaggerated emphasis on somatological and physiological processes, which have become the criteria by which pathological manifestations of an illness or its symptoms are evaluated. Extensive research (particularly experimentation with animals) has produced many new healing methods and hundreds of medications for the treatment of human illnesses. The result has been the development of enormously successful treatments for acute infections and for illnesses that can be treated surgically. On the other hand, in spite of these improvements in modern medicine, the treatment of chronic and psychosomatic illnesses remains unsatisfactory. Patients with such illnesses who are treated according to modern medical methods often suffer more from the side effects of long-term medication than from the illness itself.

Ayurveda developed over centuries as a holistic medical system. From a scientific point of view, ayurveda medicine, practised from about 1500 B.C. to 500 A.D., was remarkably advanced. The different specialties of ayurveda are comparable to those of modern medicine of the last hundred years.

In contrast to modern medicine, which primarily developed along therapeutic concepts, ayurveda addresses the basic needs of a human being on three levels. According to ayurveda, defined as "the knowledge or science of life," this concept has three components: (1) prevention,

(2) awareness of the origin of life, and (3) systematic approach for establishing the diagnosis of an illness and treatment in accordance with a medical protocol.

Tridosha (the theory of the three basic individual constitutions—*vata, pitta,* and *kapha*) is a concept that has been clinically tested and proven to be effective for centuries. Even if a precise translation of *tridosha* according to today's scientific terminology is difficult, it is viewed as representing very basic psychophysiological processes in the human body. This division into three constitutions makes sense when we realize that in ayurveda, the human organism is first viewed as an inseparable whole before an examination of its organs and systems takes place.

One of the interesting aspects of ayurveda is that the different therapies (including herbal and mineral medications) are very deliberately and very specifically correlated to the basic components of *tridosha.* In other words, they are mutually dependent so that, in a given case, an antagonistic and, therefore, stabilizing influence on the *tridoshas* can be achieved. This concept is important, because medications that are correlated almost never create negative side effects in the human body, presumably because the organism does not perceive them as foreign bodies.

Hans H. Rhyner presents the ayurvedic concept in classical style, outlining first the underlying philosophy, then moving on to the pathophysiological aspects, and concluding with a discussion of the different therapies. The author explains the typology of the different constitutions. This is followed by an extensive discussion of nutrition, including a commentary on what constitutes a healthy day in the life of a person. The latter concept has important implications for today's society with all its different forms of stress, the many negative environmental influences and their consequences, and the dangers created by the deterioration of the social norm and order. Integrating preventive and therapeutic approaches to illnesses is particularly important today, in light of the explosion of health-care costs.

Including ayurvedic medicine in the health-care system should not be viewed as competition, but as an effective addition for the treatment of chronic and psychosomatic illnesses where modern medicine is only marginally successful. This book is useful for physicians and for people who are generally interested in ayurvedic healing methods. It might also serve as an impetus for research into the basic concepts, such as *tridosha,* and of specific therapeutic methods, such as *panchakarma.* The pathophysiological concept of ayurveda clearly relates to the functional process of stress and the way it affects the immune system. An active cooperation between ayurveda and modern medicine and the natural sciences would benefit the healthy as well as the sick person. A first step in this direction

6

is already in progress with the establishment of the scientifically oriented Ayurveda Clinic in Walzenhausen, Switzerland, where the diagnostic aspects of modern medicine are being correlated with the results of ayurvedic therapy.

P. Vishwanath Rai, M.D.
Neurology, Psychiatry, Tropical Medicine, and Ayurveda

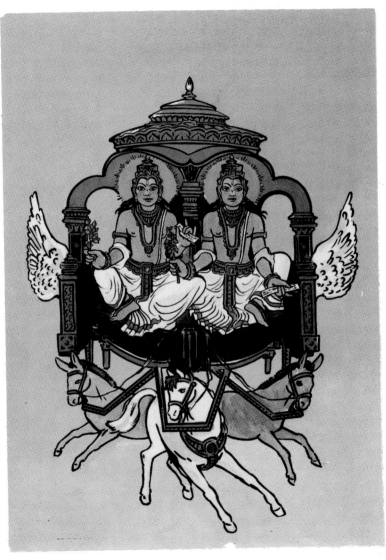

The *Ashwini* twins, divine physicians

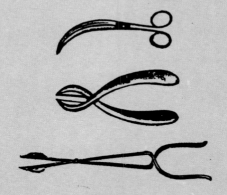

नखशस्त्रम् ।

वक्रार्जुधारं द्विमुखं नखशस्त्रं नवाङ्गुलम् ।
सूक्ष्मशस्त्रोद्धृतिच्छेदभेदप्रच्छानलेखने ॥

दन्तलेखनम् ।

एकधारं चतुष्कोणं प्रवृद्धग्राकृति चैकतः ।
दन्तलेखनकं तेन शोधयेद्दन्तशर्करान् ॥

सूची ।

वृत्ता गूढतृढाः पार्श्वे तिस्रः सूच्योत्र सीवने ।
मांसलानां प्रदेशानां वृत्ता त्र्यङ्गुलमायता ॥
षष्ठमांसास्थिसन्धिस्थव्रणानां द्व्यङ्गुलायता ।
त्रीह्निवक्रा धनुर्वक्रा पक्षामाग्ग्यमर्म्मसु ॥
सा सार्द्धत्र्यङ्गुला सर्व्वी वृत्ताद्याः सूचयः स्मृताः ॥

Instruments used by Susruta, in the Vinod Lal Sengupta's book
Ayurveda-Vijnanam (Calcutta, 1929)

Ayurveda, the Mother of Medicine
Ithihasa

History and Legend

Ayurveda is the science of life. Its origin is closely related to the cultural development that has taken place over the centuries, and it continues to be influenced by them. *Ayurveda* comes from two Sanskrit words, *ayus,* meaning "life," and *veda,* meaning "wisdom" or "science." Ayurveda has never been shrouded in mystery. Its unorthodox philosophy, containing some elements of atheism, has its roots in the matriarchal teachings of the Tantra—that's why we use the feminine form throughout this book. This philosophy, consistent with the ancient Indian understanding of ayurveda, gives it utmost flexibility and has helped make ayurveda part of the Chinese, Tibetan, Greek, and Arabic cultures. Ayurveda, considered the "mother of medicine," has spread throughout the world in many different forms.

In ancient times, wise men gathered in consultation, sharing their experiences in the many different branches of science. Important discoveries, conclusions, and even disagreements were carefully recorded. Some of these wise men (whose purpose in life was to maintain the well-being of everything living on earth) possessed extraordinary powers of contemplation, which gave them the ability to understand reality in terms of its most minute, interrelated processes.

Over time, as a result of these meetings, six philosophical systems (*darshanas*) evolved. These included the study of logic (*nyaya*), the theory of the atom (*vaiseshika*), the thesis of evolution and the axiom of causality (*sankhya*), the discipline of body and spirit (*yoga*), moral behavior (*mimasa*), and pure, esoteric knowledge (*vedanta*), all of which are part of ayurveda.

One attains wisdom through *sruti,* which literally means "to have heard something without another person present." We would call this "direct revelation." Such "knowing" is part of every culture. This process also has its place in the natural sciences, where researchers, after years of

9

intensive work, suddenly find the solution or answer, which is not really new but has existed all along. *Veda* and *upanisha* are part of the *srutis*. In contrast, *smritis* is the body of knowledge that is passed on from master to student. *Puranas, ramayana, mahabharata, vedangas, sutras,* and *dharmashastra* are part of *smritis*. Although ayurveda is considered part of the *atharvaveda,* it has developed a consistent, separate philosophy. Clearly, it has nothing to do with so-called primitive mentality or magical rituals, which is quite remarkable, considering how long ayurveda has been practised.

In Indian legend, Atreya, a vedic wise man and author of the fifth book of *Rigveda,* was the first human being the gods taught the art of medicine. The traditional council of wise men could no longer watch an increasing number of illnesses befall animals and humans. Atreya was chosen to learn about ayurveda from these higher beings.

Devtas, or gods, are beings who resemble humans but have a life expectancy much greater than that of ordinary humans. They have specific abilities, due to the composition of their bodies. Atreya took on a different dimension and went to see Indra, the king of the gods. Important personalities are said to have been travelling on flying machines or in the form of astral bodies, throughout the galaxy. Atreya also gave a report about the relativity of time on other planets. For instance, Mucukunda, who spent extended periods of time in higher planetary systems and who participated in intergalactic wars, found none of his family members alive when he returned to Earth, because, in his absence, many thousands of Earth years had passed.

Atreya spoke to the king of the gods, "Oh, monarch of the gods, not only do you reign over the heavenly spheres but over all three planetary systems, because that is the way the Creator wanted it. The world of the human beings is befallen with illnesses, and they suffer terribly. Show your compassion and teach me the science of life."

After Indra had convinced himself of Atreya's brilliant intellectual capabilities, he taught the wise man about ayurveda, which he himself had received from two physicians, the divine Ashwini brothers. The Ashwini brothers had received their knowledge from Daksha, who had the task of filling the universe with living beings. Daksha had been instructed by his father Brahma, the first living being of the universe.

Atreya, the most outstanding among the wise men, recorded what he learned. He passed the records on to the following students: Agnivesha, Bhela, Jatukarna, Parasara, Ksirapani, and Harita. Each student added his own commentary. The writings of Agnivesha, the *Caraka-Samhita,* have survived, practically intact, while the books written by Bhela and Harita exist only in fragments. These texts describe, for the first time, the eight different disciplines of ayurveda (*astanga ayurveda*).

These disciplines include Indian versions of general medicine, pediatrics, psychiatry, ears-nose-throat and ophthalmic specialties, surgery, toxicology, geriatrics, and sex studies. In addition to these eight disciplines, ayurveda includes extensive knowledge of veterinary medicine.

Kaya-cikitsa (general medicine) describes research into the causes, symptoms, healing methods, and therapeutic interventions for most illnesses.

Bala-cikitsa or *kaumarabhritya* (pediatrics) deals with the illnesses of children.

Bhuta-vidya or *graha-cikitsa* (psychiatry) is the science of psychological disturbances and mental illness.

Urdhvanga-cikitsa or *salakya* (ears-nose-throat and ophthalmology) deals with the ears, nose, throat, and eyes. It also describes minor surgery of organs located above the collarbone.

Salya-tantra (surgery) is the science of treating organs with pathological disturbances and changes in the organism.

Agada-tantra (toxicology) studies poisons and poisoned organisms.

Rasayana (geriatrics) is the science of aging.

Vajikarana (sexology) is the study of sex.

Ayurveda Training

Modern ayurveda training pays close attention to the original teachings and how they developed over time. Students have always had a choice of studying in any of three different ways. They could live and work directly with a master, enroll in a school, living and studying with other students and a teacher or master (these schools were usually located in remote areas), or enroll in a university (located in large cities, such as Taxila, Kashi, Vidaha, or Nalanda). These universities have attracted students from all over the world since the seventh century A.D.

The University of Taxila, near what is known today as Rawalpindi in Pakistan, enjoyed great fame because of its excellent medical school. Historically verified records about this school still exist. Some were written by Plinus, Strabo, and historians accompanying Alexander the Great on his journey to India. Famous scientists, such as Panini, Jivaka, Bhikshu, Vyadi, Nagarjuna, Deva, Brahmadatta, and Junaha, studied at this university or were closely connected to it.

11

Another well-known center of learning was Nalanda, near the city known today as Bihar. Here, the study of ayurveda was obligatory. The university flourished from the fifth to the twelfth century. People such as Hiuent Sung and I Tsing came from China to study. The campus covered more than ⅔ square mile (1 sq km). The facilities included eight large halls, some six stories high, and 300 lecture halls. The library was housed in three large buildings. More than 1,500 professors and 10,000 students inhabited the city. Clothes, meals, and housing were free; expenses were paid by kings and well-to-do citizens.

Kashi, today called Benares, was another very famous institute of learning. It specialized in surgery. *Salakya,* the ears, nose, and throat specialty, was taught primarily in Vihada under Nimi. Several faculties in southern India taught *rasashastra* (the production of medication from minerals) and toxicology.

Invasions, beginning in the Middle Ages and lasting for centuries, destroyed practically every university. British invaders brought with them modern Western medicine and quickly began to establish their own universities. That ayurveda survived at all is due solely to the master-student tradition. Not until the first Indian revolution in 1857 (the British still refer to it as The Great Mutiny), did it become clear to the people of India how important it was to preserve their own social and cultural traditions. The same revolutionary spirit led to the establishment of the Indian Congress, which affirmed its support of ayurvedic medicine. As late as 1917, an application for the establishment of an ayurvedic university was rejected by the British government, which recognized only modern Western medicine as legitimate. It wasn't until February 13, 1921, that Mahatma Gandhi was able to open the Tibbi College for Ayurveda and Unani Medicine in Delhi; others followed soon thereafter.

Today, India has approximately 55 state and 70 private universities and learning institutions where ayurvedic medicine is taught. The government requires that every university and every college have a university hospital. Sri Lanka, Nepal, Malaysia, Indonesia, Bangladesh, and Pakistan all have similar institutions.

The study of ayurvedic medicine takes 11 semesters. It is also possible to earn a doctorate in several specialty areas. More than 2,000 dissertations and research papers are housed in different state institutions, attesting to the new surge of inquiry into this ancient science.

Classic Ayurveda Textbooks

Ayurveda can look with pride to a rich treasure of classical medical literature. Remarkably, some of the almost 3,500-year-old works are still used as official textbooks. Among others, the Great Trilogy (*Brihat Trayi*) occupies a prominent place. This trilogy consists of the *Caraka-Samhita, Susruta-Samhita,* and *Astanga-Samgraha.*

Brihat Trayi

Caraka-Samhita

This volume is the oldest purely medical text. Although the original manuscripts have been lost, we still have access to their content. At least four authors contributed to this volume. The first was Atreya, followed by his immediate student Agnivesha; later, different and incomplete copies were collected by Dridhabala and Caraka and combined in one volume. *Caraka-Samhita* has been divided into eight parts (*sthanas*), and these, in turn, are divided into different chapters.

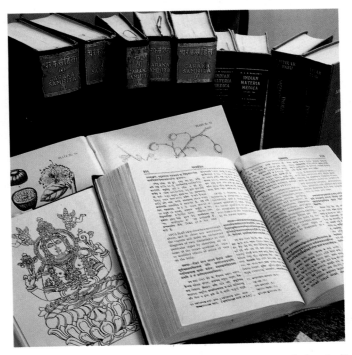

The first English edition of the *Caraka-Samhita* (1949), and the *Indian Materia Medica* (1908) by Nadkarnis.

Sutra-Sthanam, the first book, is a compilation of material. It begins with an introduction to health, medicine, hygiene, prophylaxis, diet, and life-style. This is followed by a list of the four components necessary for successful treatment—the physician, the medication, the patient, and the nurse. Oil and sweat therapies and the cause of the illness are discussed.

13

There is also advice on how to build a hospital. Atreya remarks that a person hit by lightning has a better chance of survival than a patient who falls into the hands of a quack.

Nidana-Sthanam, the second book, deals with the pathology of eight serious diseases—fever, bleeding, tumors and ulcers, urinary tract diseases, skin diseases, general physical deterioration of the body or of individual organs, and epilepsy. Each illness is discussed individually. Its cause, manifestation, extent, diagnostic aids, and treatment are examined in detail.

Vimana-Sthanam, the third book, deals with chemistry, physiology, anatomy, epidemiology, infectious diseases, the three ways of arriving at a diagnosis (observation, inference, and questioning), diseases of the circulatory, digestive, and elimination systems, parasitic illnesses, and different ways of teaching medical students. When Agnivesha asked what the terms *timely* and *untimely death* mean, because every person had an undetermined life expectancy, Atreya answered that a perfect axle on a car will wear out naturally over time. In the same way, the life span of a human being will be used up, and the person will die naturally. However, the wear and tear on the axle will be that much greater if the load of the wagon is increased, an unqualified driver is driving the wagon, the roads are bad, maintenance is poor, and so forth. In the same way, the life expectancy of a person will be shortened when the person is under constant stress; when food cannot be properly digested; when meals are irregular; when body posture is poor; when sexual activities are too frequent; when a natural life-style is repressed; when a person indulges in an unhealthy life-style; when microorganisms invade the body; when the air is polluted; when a person is injured, eats the wrong food, or takes the wrong medication; and when improper medical manipulations are carried out.

Sharira-Sthanam, the fourth book, covers human anatomy, reproduction and pregnancies, the development of the fetus in the mother's womb, and the role of the mother's milk. It even discusses toys and amulets for the newborn.

Indriya-Sthanam, the fifth book, covers symptomatology, diagnosis, and prognosis. A large portion deals with signs that indicate that a patient is near death.

Cikitsa-Sthanam, the sixth book, is the most important for practising physicians, because it describes many therapies and medications.

Kalpha-Sthanam, the seventh book, deals with a great number of for-

14

mulas and medications that induce vomiting or have laxative properties.

Siddhi-Sthanam, the eighth book, deals with ayurveda's classical method of detoxification, called *panchakarma.*

The *Caraka-Samhita* contains 341 recipes made from plants, 177 medications using animal products, and 64 medications using minerals and metals. The work was translated into Arabic, and a little later, in the eighth century, into Persian by Ali-ibn-Zain from Tarbistan. The term *sharaka indianus* can also be found in the Latin translation of Rhazes (680 A.D.) and Avicenna.

Susruta-Samhita

This book describes the tradition of surgery in Indian medicine. The author is believed to be the scholar Sustruta, who lived over 3,000 years ago. *Susruta-Samhita* is considered one of the four principal books on surgery and the only work still existing today, though not in its original form. The roots of the work have been traced directly to Dhanvantari (the incarnation of Vishnu), who is said to have been Susruta's teacher. Every chapter begins with the words, *"Vathovaca bhagavan Dhanvantari Susrutaya,"* or, "As Susruta was taught by the 'honorable *Dhanvantari'."* *Dhanvantariyas,* as surgeons were called then, were already known during Caraka's time.

Susruta-Samhita consists of six books (the last is an appendix that was added later) and 184 chapters. This classic work on surgery is probably the most important of its kind. It remains unknown to the medical profession in Europe and America to this day, although an English translation by Hoernle and Kunte was published in 1876. Many modern Western scientists did not accept the fact that gunpowder was discovered long ago in the East. However, it appears that the same scientists who dismissed ayurveda also copied freely from its writings.

The *Susruta-Samhita* describes 76 eye conditions, 51 of which were treated surgically. The author counts 101 blunt and 20 sharp surgical instruments that are surprisingly similar to the instruments used today. The human hand, the most important instrument, is included in this count.

Surgical intervention was used in a very restricted sense, and only when other treatments could not promise success. *Susruta* distinguishes among eight different types of surgery.

Incision (cutting) for deep abscesses, erysipelas, swollen testicles, carbuncles, ulcers, and fistulas
Excision (removing tissues) for anal fistulas, moles, edges of wounds,

tumors, growths, ulcers, and foreign objects in bones or muscles

Scarification (incisions that extract blood or fluids) used for throat infections, leukocytes, and ulcers on the surface of the tongue

Puncture (with a hollow needle) to extract fluids from diseased veins and from the tunica vaginalis of the testicles, and for dropsy

Sounding Out (with a probe) for poorly healing wounds and wounds in which foreign objects are imbedded

Extraction (surgical removal) for removing foreign objects, tartar from the teeth, and removal of a dead fetus from the womb

Evacuation (removing fluids) used in cases of localized swelling, blood poisoning, pustules, abscesses, and leprosylike skin diseases

Suture (closure of wound or incision) to close open wounds and joint injuries

In addition to simple surgical procedures, more complex operations, such as plastic surgery, skin transplants, and amputations, were also performed.

Patients were usually anesthetized, but the methods used then could not be used today, although some were described in sufficient detail for duplication (such as the inhalation of particular drugs to induce sleep or to regain consciousness). However, we do know of several healing plants with antibiotic properties that prevent infections after surgery.

Just as today, medical students practised their surgical skills on corpses. However, at that time, the practice was strictly forbidden by Buddhism, which was the beginning of the end of ayurvedic surgery. The problem

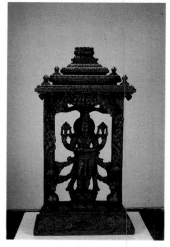

Sculpture of Dhanvantari, the patron of physicians and patients

during ancient times was much as it is today—when financial support for research institutions is cut, the possibility of active research is reduced and the subject of the research disappears. We should not be surprised then, that ayurvedic surgery, without any research support for 2,000 years, disappeared. Only in this century have Indian universities tried again to combine surgical science and medicine. For instance, at the University of Benares, future ayurvedic physicians are required to study modern surgery.

Susruta-Samhita discusses 1,120 illnesses, including injuries, illnesses relating to aging, and mental illness. These discussions include 700 healing plants, 57 preparations derived from animal sources, and 64 prepa-

16

rations derived from minerals. Around 800 A.D., Ibn Abillsaibial translated the *Susruta-Samhita* into Arabic under the title *Kitabshah-shun-al-hindi.*

Astanga-Samgraha

This is the last and most recent volume of the three main books. A Chinese pilgrim, I-Tsing, wrote around 500 A.D. that the earlier works of Indian medicine had been combined by Vagbhata into one new volume. Vagbhata was born in Sindh (a province in Pakistan) and was taught ayurvedic medicine by his father and a Buddhist monk, named Avalokita. Historians still argue about a correct date, and the numbers fluctuate anywhere from 200 B.C. to 500 A.D. From his notes, we can assume that Vagbhata was a Buddhist. Because of his religion, his work found its way to Tibet and from there to China and Japan.

Vagbhata was the first author who mentioned the concept of medical astrology in his writings. He wrote that the course of illnesses, if they occur under different astrological constellations, take different turns. His compilation, *Astanga-Samgraha,* consists of six volumes and 16 chapters. The word *astanga* suggests that this work deals with the eightfold concept of ayurveda (*astanga-ayurveda*).

The **first book** of the *Astanga-Samgraha* consists of 40 chapters. It is an excellent introduction to the subject. Here, the author discusses health, a long life free of sickness, personal hygiene (a subject that universities in European medical schools did not include until the end of the nineteenth century), the causes of illness, how times of the day or year influence the human organism, types and classifications of medicine, the significance of the sense of taste, bio-energies, therapies, surgical intervention, and phlebotomy.

The **second book** has 12 chapters. This volume describes human anatomy, pregnancy and possible complications during birth, individual constitutions, and various aids for establishing a prognosis.

The **third book** has 16 chapters. It discusses diagnostics and pathology.

The **fourth book** has 24 chapters. It describes the treatment of illnesses discussed in the previous book.

The **fifth book** has 8 chapters. This book deals with therapies, such as therapeutically induced vomiting, the use of laxatives, enemas, complications that might occur during such therapies, and the necessary medications.

The **sixth book** has 50 chapters. It presents the most detailed work of *Astanga-Samgraha,* filling in details not discussed in the previous books.

The author wrote another famous book, *Astanga-Hridaya,* which is a condensed version of the *Astanga Samgraha*. This work is particularly favored because of the clarity of its presentation. We know of the existence of 37 commentaries, early Tibetan and Arabic translations, as well as a German translation by L. Hilgenberg and W. Kirfel, published in 1937 in Leiden. The first complete English translation of the *Astanga-Samgraha* is in progress, undertaken by Professor M. Mahadeva Shastry at the International Ayurveda Research Center in Bangalore. This work is immense in scope and requires an extensive knowledge of Sanskrit and medicine.

Laghu Trayi

Among the many texts about ayurveda, three works hold a prominent place, the Small Trilogy (*Laghu Trayi*).

Madhava Nidana

Madhava, an important author, wrote the *Roga Viniscaya* around 700 A.D. Better known as the *Madhava Nidina*, this book is very popular and much referred to in pathology. It talks about the causes of illnesses, pathology, symptomatology, and prognosis, but it does not suggest treatments. Less than 50 years after it was written, the caliph Harun-al-Rashid ordered it translated into Arabic. Mario Vallduri translated five chapters into Italian under the title *Saggio de versione del madhava nidana*. The manuscript was published in Florence in 1914 by the Giornale della Societa Asiatica Italiana. G. J. Meulenbeld made the first English translation under the title of *The Madhava Nidana and Its Chief Commentary* (published in 1974 by E. J. Brill for the Orientalo-Rheno-Traiectina in Leiden).

Sarangadhara-Samhita

The second book of this trilogy was written around 1226. The author, Sarangadhara, explains that it was supposed to be a handbook for the practicing physician. In the first part, he discusses terminology, weights and measurements, when herbs for medicinal purposes should be harvested, definitions of pharmacological terms, pulse diagnosis, and much more. The second part deals with proportions and the preparation of medications. In the last part, he discusses different therapies, such as oil and sweat therapy, inhalations, gargling, phlebotomy, and so forth.

Sarangadhara was the first Indian author to: (1) use the pulse diagnosis (*nadi pariksha*) as a diagnostic tool, (2) discuss the mechanism of oxygen exchange, (3) establish clear pharmacological terminology, (4) include opium and other healing substances in his *Materia Medica*, (5) mention that medications can be administered directly into the bloodstream via an artificial wound (injection), and (6) provide a description

18

of dracontiasis (an illness caused by the guinea worm, the longest thread-worm that lives in the human body). His therapy is still the only means by which this horrible parasite, which can grow up to a yard (1 m) long, can be totally removed.

Not until 1984 was this work translated into English by K. R. Srikanta Murthy.

Bhava-Prakasa

This, the latest volume, was written by Bhava Misra in 1558. Considered the standard text in medicine, it deals with the concepts of causation, symptoms, and cures of illnesses. In this book, the lists of illnesses and treatments were brought up to date; for instance, syphilis, which reached India when the Portuguese merchant marines began arriving on the subcontinent, is mentioned for the first time.

Modern Medicine and the Possibilities of Ayurveda

The use of ayurveda offers many possibilities in our time. Even though modern medicine has made great strides, cures for many illnesses and sufferings remain illusive, particularly those affecting the metabolism, systemic illnesses (affecting the whole organism), and psychosomatic illnesses. For centuries, ayurvedic medicine has provided proven treat-ments for chronic illnesses. Since ayurveda looks at health and illness in a holistic way and considers the patient's specific qualities and person-ality as well as the sociocultural environment in which he lives, the treatments developed can be employed anywhere, anytime. Skepticism and concerns that ayurveda is not suitable for individuals living in the Western world can be put aside. We might add that for hundreds of years, if not for centuries, ayurveda has made valuable contributions to our understanding of medicine—knowledge that came to us through Greek, Roman, and Greco-Arabic cultures.

Ayurvedic terms for illnesses and diagnoses have been translated into the languages of modern medicine. The use of ayurvedic treatment meth-ods, therefore, is easy in cases where modern allopathic medicine con-tinues to be unsuccessful or does not achieve the desired result. In many cases, ayurvedic medications and therapies can be combined with ongo-ing treatments that use chemical, pharmaceutical, or homeopathic med-ications, since ayurvedic preparations do not create any negative side effects. Ayurvedic healing methods, therefore, can be used even if other treatment methods have been tried in the past.

The ever-increasing number of chronic illnesses and the explosion of health-care costs should be reason enough for physicians and politicians alike to examine the many different therapeutic possibilities that the implementation of ayurvedic medicine offers. A first step in this direction would be to present such alternatives in continuing education courses for physicians and to establish research programs that should be made available to nonmedical scientists. The public is asking for new, more natural treatment methods that do not create side effects. In the long run, people will not be deterred by the resistance voiced by modern physicians.

According to ayurveda, life expectancy for a human being is about 100 years. We have the right to spend these years in good health and in full possession of all our mental faculties. Ayurveda has given us the means by which to reach this goal. It gives us an understanding of the connection between body, mind, and soul, offering advice for a more natural, healthy life-style, pointing out how important discipline is in our professional and personal lives. It also shows us how to normalize the metabolic process through proper diet and a properly functioning autonomic system and how to stimulate the body's own healing powers.

Philosophical and Medical Basis
Adisthana Tattva

Applying the Principles of Six Classical, Philosophical Systems

Like every other natural science, ayurveda uses existing hypotheses to define structure, effect, and other characteristics of its subject. The holistic and pragmatic approach ayurveda uses is extraordinary. It integrates six classical systems of thought—*sankhya*, yoga, *nyaya, vaisheshika, vedanta*, and *mimasa*. The names might sound strange, but their basic principles can be applied to every philosophical, religious, and scientific system.

Sankhya philosophy explains important principles, such as those of the five elements, three "omni-substances," and three "bio-energies." *Sankhya*, an analytical system, reduces a substance to its primary matter, and all reduce nature to the two basic opposing principles—matter and antimatter. Most scientists have this understanding, but employ it only in a general way. *Sankhya* goes further to examine spirit, intelligence, and ego, as well as antimatter. Human beings, animals, and plants are seen as a microcosm of the universe; the only differences are in quantity and relative proportions. Just as a painter can create endless color combinations from three different basic colors, so every human being, plant, and animal is a unique, individual whole in this universe.

Six Systems of Ayurvedic Thought

Sankhya	Thesis of evolution
Yoga	Discipline of body and spirit
Nyaya	Logic
Vaisheshika	Science of atoms
Vedanta	Esoterica
Mimasa	Responsibility and reward

Basic Elements According to *Sankhya* Philosophy

Antimatter

Purusha, or antimatter, remains unaltered and consists of pure consciousness. It is without form, cannot be divided, does not occupy space, and often is referred to as the male principle. Antimatter may be called the spark of life, or "bio." In other words, it is the principle which constitutes the difference between those bodies or cells that are lifeless and those that are alive. A dead person certainly consists of the same physical components as a person who is alive. Bones, brain, heart, lungs, blood, nerves, bone marrow, and skin are still present. Nothing disappears after the person dies. Some cells, such as those of the hair and nails, even continue to grow. What then disappears? Only consciousness, the sign of antimatter. Even on the atomic and subatomic level, antimatter is the driving force. Nuclear physicists verify this and also use the term *antimatter*. This minute spark of antimatter fills the universe with countless living beings (just as the flame of one single candle can light countless others) and, in harmony with ur-matter, can take on unlimited numbers of shapes and colors.

25 Basic Elements According to Classical *Sankhya* Philosophy

Purusha (antimatter)   Elemental and individual consciousness (the soul)
Prakriti (ur-matter)   If omni-substances *sattva, rajas,* and *tamas* are not visible = *avyakta;* when *sattva, rajas,* and *tamas* are visible = *vyakta*
Ahankara (ego)
Buddhi (intelligence)
Manas (psyche)
Tanmaras (five senses)   Sound, touch, sight, taste, and smell
Pancamahabhuta (five elements)   Ether, air, fire, water, and earth
Jnanendriyas (five sense organs)   Ears, skin, eyes, tongue, and nose
Karmendriyas (five action organs)   Speech, handling, locomotion, evacuation, and reproduction

Ur-Matter

Prakriti, or ur-matter, is the growing medium for all physical and chemical processes in the universe. When leaving its nonmanifest, original

22

state, an evolutionary process is set in motion which creates 23 cosmic key principles. The quantity is unchangeable. Ur-matter is compressed to its basic form or, when expanding, initiates the whole process of creation. The potential for this explosion resides within the process. The trigger for the evolutionary process is the enormous tensions between matter and antimatter.

Omni-Substance

Ur-matter can be divided into three specific omni-substances (*trigunas*). As long as the balance between the omni-substances is not disturbed, they remain in their preevolutionary state (*avyakta*). Depending on the amount of tension between ur-matter and antimatter and its effect, omni-substances lose their balance. The light substance (*sattva*) remains closer to the antimatter, the more inert substance (*tamas*) closer to the ur-matter, and the dynamic substance (*rajas*) remains in the center of the field of tension.

Omni-substances influence the interplay of forces between matter. From miniscule to very coarse structure, an ever-increasing density and differentiation of the ur-matter takes place. No one is able to imagine a huge, widely branched tree when looking at a small seed, although that is how it will manifest itself over time. Similarly, the whole evolutionary process of creation is present in ur-matter, beginning at the level of microparticles.

Ego

No matter how coarse or physically large a process (reaction) seems to be, in the final analysis, everything starts at the micro level. For example, hundreds of streetcars roll through a large city and countless lights illuminate the streets. Yet with one flick of a switch at the electrical power station, everything comes to a standstill. If we pursue this line of reasoning, we know that certain mental processes were at work before the switch was turned off, including a "yes" or "no" decision. This decision and the location of the switch are the equivalents of the microstructures of ego.

Intelligence

Buddhi, or intelligence, is one of the internal cognitive instruments that allow us to create an image of the specific characteristics of an object. Parts of the functioning of the basic substance are perception (awareness), cognition, memory, rationality, and the ability to think in the abstract. Factors that can interfere with the normal functions of recognition are grief, anger, passion, ridicule, envy, jealousy, doubt, horror, and capriciousness.

Psyche

Manas, or psyche, consists of microparticles that, developing to the next phase, contain the five coarse-structured elements—ether, air fire, water, and earth. The element of air is dominant in the psyche, which makes it possible to measure brain currents. Spirit cannot be detected by sense organs, only by itself. The seat of the spirit is the thalamus, or *ajna chakra*. Every human body has one psyche, and this psyche is inseparable from the body for life. The psyche receives impulses from the cognitive organs (*jnanendriyas*) and passes them on to the tactile senses. However, the psyche is also able to mentally register objects normally outside the perception of the senses (*indriyas*). This ability is called the 11th sense (5 sense organs + 5 tactile organs + psyche = 11). It distinguishes between the characteristics of perception and action and is known as the super sense, because every object of the other senses is also the object of the 11th sense, which regulates and activates all senses.

Sense organs alone can only observe nonrestricted data, which the psyche uses to solve problems. Functions of the psyche independent of the senses include the fulfillment of dreams, cognition, consideration, reasoning, imagination, feelings, and will.

The psyche can be viewed as threefold (*trividham*)—pure (*sattvik*), hyperactive (*rajasik*), and sluggish (*tamasik*). It is related to the three omni-substances *sattva*, *rajas*, and *tamas*. For this reason, the omni-substances are also called bio-energies (*manasa dosha*) in ayurveda. While bodily disturbances can develop when the three bio-energies are out of balance, only *rajas* and *tamas* can induce illnesses of the psyche, because by nature the psyche is *sattvik*.

In *sattva*, body and spirit are in a state of minimal positive activity. *Rajas*, on the other hand, stimulates the psyche, which can disturb the balance, pulling a person out of lethargy. During the course of a day, every human being and every animal is in an aggressive state, which apparently leads to endless activity. Under this influence, all living beings, and human beings in particular, cling to their world. *Rajas* is the root of all suffering. *Tamas* is the negative quality of *sattva* and *rajas*. Since the psyche in *tamas* withdraws from *sattva* and *rajas*, it becomes unable to react to normal stimuli.

Psyche and body are closely connected to each other. Mental activities are manifest through the body. On the other hand, the body gives the psyche the necessary nutrition. The dominant quality of the way we live, therefore, will always have an effect on the psyche. For that reason,

24

ayurveda classifies food into *sattvik, rajasik,* and *tamasik* (see also the chapter Nutritional Science, under "General Rules"). In conclusion, we can say that ego, intelligence, and psyche represent the microstructure of body. Each of these three basic substances has definite, individual, and original characteristics which enable us to arrive at a comprehensible holistic picture of a human being. This consistent analytical approach used by ayurveda is particularly valuable in psychiatry. Mental physiology is seen from a whole new perspective, which allows for unheard-of therapeutic possibilities.

The Senses

"In the beginning was the Word." So it is written in the *Book of All Books* and in other writings which have served as the basis for every world religion. Even if we start, as some scientists do, with the not so imaginative big-bang theory, creation is said to have begun with a huge explosion. The *sankhya* philosophy distinguishes between elements that are still invisible, expressing themselves through their sound, texture, color, shape, taste, and smell, and those that are visible. This would be one way of solving the age-old riddle of which came first, the chicken or the egg? First, there is the chicken in the invisible form, but with all its qualities in place. It then becomes slowly visible via the elementary parts of the egg.

The Elements

Sound waves need space (ether) in order to expand. The element ether is set in motion and condenses to become air. The constant movement of air and its density leads to friction, which leads to the next condensed element, fire, with its quality of color and shape. The heat of the fire condenses water, which has the quality of taste. A solid mass, earth, is formed when water cools down. This has the quality of smell.

Ether has just one quality—sound. Each element that follows has the quality of the one that preceded it, which means that *air* also has sound and density; *fire* consists of sound, density, shape, and color; *water* has sound, density, color, and taste; and *earth* has sound, density, shape, color, taste, and its own, unique quality of smell.

The words *ether, air, fire, water,* and *earth* are often misunderstood. They are not connected to and do not correspond with the Sanskrit terms *akasha, vayu, tejas, ap,* and *prithivi.* Air includes all gaslike elements and combinations. Brilliance, heat, color, and shape are all part of fire. All liquid substances point to the element of water. Everything solid has elements of earth. Ether occupies the largest space, since its atomic particles are very loosely arranged. Earth, on the other hand, takes the least amount of space, since its atomic particles are very densely arranged. Whenever a reduction or expansion of these elements takes place, energy is either used or created.

In ayurveda, the theory of the elements has nothing in common with that of the Greeks or Romans (who only knew four elements), or, for that matter, has it anything in common with modern physics, which has over 100 elements. The view on this subject, therefore, is consistent with the overall approach, as we can see from the following examples.

In ayurveda, just as in nuclear physics, a void does not consist of emptiness; rather, it is made up of the most minute substances. Physicists have removed all air from a particle accelerator through a vacuum pump, cooled this void to absolute zero, and initiated acceleration. They found that particles were still present. These microparticles are called *akasha* (in ayurveda), ether, or space. Normally, we do not find such elements in pure form in nature. By establishing the characteristics of an object, we are able to define the most dominant element. The table on which I may be sitting is solid, hard, and heavy. Thus, the predominant element is earth. The pillow on which I am sitting, thanks to the presence of air and space, feels soft and light.

About 150 years ago, the English physicist and chemist John Dalton (1766–1844) declared that the atom was the smallest particle and could not be divided any further. Since that time, this theory has had to be revised, because as we now know, atoms can and have been split. From

Basic Composition of the Sense of Taste

Taste	Composition
Tangy	Air and earth
Bitter	Air and ether
Sharp	Air and fire
Salty	Water and fire
Sour	Earth and fire
Sweet	Earth and water

the ayurvedic point of view, even an atom consists of five elements. Its weight comes from the element *earth,* its cohesion from the element *water,* its energy from the element *fire,* the motion of its subatomic particles around the nucleus from the element *air,* and the spaces between its particles from the element *ether.*

Although the human body consists primarily of water and earth, we also find all the other elements. All hollow spaces, such as the throat, trachea, esophagus, sinuses, and ear canals, consist of the element ether. The air in the lungs, vessels, and pores within the bones all consist of the

Characteristics of Elements and Their Effects

Element	Characteristic	Effect
Ether (*akasha*)	Light, fine, smooth, soft	Porous, soft, and producing lightness
Air (*vayu*)	Light, cold, dry, rough, fine	Activating, stimulating motion, stimulating lightness and roughness
Fire (*tejas*)	Hot, sharp, fine, light, dry, clear	Stimulating digestion, supporting the aura, producing heat
Water (*ap*)	Liquid, oily, cold, slow, soft, mucous	Moistening, holding together, dissolving
Earth (*prithivi*)	Heavy, coarse, hard, slow, stabile, solid, rough, clear	Stimulating growth, stabilizing, strengthening, supporting compactness

element air. The whole digestive tract, representing a kind of fire, consists of the element fire.

Each individual represents a unique combination of these elements and their homeostasis, which means self-regulation of the individual biological system. What will cure one individual might make another sick. But this is true not only for the human body, which consists of all five elements, but also for all plants, animals, and minerals, as well as all the solid, liquid, and gaseous materials around us. An excess of one or more elements can be the cause of illnesses and of a disturbance of natural balance. Substances that are able to reestablish homeostasis are not all that difficult to find. Ayurveda has worked out a simple formula.

This formula is based on the action of the three bio-energies. The thesis states that two things that are alike will strengthen each other; two opposites will weaken each other. What follows is a simple example.

Three people are hiking on a hot summer day. The constitution of each one is different, and, therefore, their temperaments are different. The person in whom the fire element is dominant is of medium build and has a hot temper. She is the one who will suffer most from the heat. The person in whom the water and earth elements are dominant is strong, plump, and good-natured. While she will perspire more easily, the heat does not bother her that much. The person in whom the elements of ether and air are dominant is slender, lean, somewhat insecure, and shy. She barely perspires and feels very comfortable in the heat. Similarly, these three people will react differently if they eat the same food or are given the same medication.

In addition to their own characteristics (*guna*), some elements also have one or more taste preferences (*raas*) which have very distinct characteristics, corresponding to their basic combinations. Each taste, or flavor, therefore, has distinct physiological effects that can be precisely defined. Pathological consequences occur when flavors are used in excess. These can be traced back to their basic composition.

Each person possesses a sense of taste that can be helpful when used with this universal analysis. The six tastes are *tangy, bitter, sharp, salty, sour,* and *sweet.* With this method of categorization, food and healing substances can be used according to how they affect the bio-energies. This subject is further discussed in the chapter Nutritional Science.

Sense and Tactile Organs

The sense and tactile organs are instruments of perception and action; they stimulate and initiate action. They have developed from the basic substance ego. *Indriya* is literally the faculty that "belongs to the master of the body."

The sense organs, *jnanendriyas* or "wisdom-collecting senses," collect impressions from the environment and pass them on to the psyche; they could be called the cognitive organs. The tactile organs, *karmendriya* or "working senses," are set in motion by orders "from the top" and are motor organs.

Three Bio-Energies (*Tridoshas*)

Although the body developed from the five elements, its creation is based on the three bio-energies—*vata, pitta,* and *kapha.* This is a concept unique to ayurveda. One might want to ask why it was necessary to establish such a concept, since the question of the body's composition has already been answered with the theory of the elements. This question can be answered by discussing ayurvedic purposes.

Ayurveda pursues two main purposes—preserving the health of an individual and healing a sick one. Every disturbance in the normal balance of the five elements creates an illness. Just as there are countless individual bodies, it follows that there are also countless illnesses. Therefore, there is no guarantee that a physician can find a particular substance that will bring a body back into balance. In addition, it is extremely difficult to determine the exact proportional shift that has taken place in the five elements and to find the countless indirect causes of an illness.

For this reason, ayurvedic physicians developed simple methods of categorizing the physiological body functions and their pathology—the three bio-energies of *vata, pitta,* and *kapha.*

Ayurveda accepts the concept that the cell is the fundamental unit, governing relatively independent biological activities (Caraka, *Sarira Sthanam*). Thus, the cell can be seen as the collective denominator of all living matter.

Even though cells have numerous functions, it is possible to reduce them to three categories or groups.

Motion—the correlative and communicative power by which one part of the body can influence another part and through which either the whole body or parts of the body can be set in motion (bio-energy *vata*)
Conversion—the substantive and metabolic power which is the cause of bio-chemical changes (bio-energy *pitta)*
Design—the nourishing and preserving powers which protect the human organism and its reproduction (bio-energy *kapha*)

The three bio-energies cannot be seen as totally separate entities, since living matter also creates an inseparable unity. However, they stand in clear and definite relation to each other. When functioning normally, they have physiological characteristics; when their function is disturbed, they have pathological characteristics. In other words, the factors of bio-energies are physiopathological.

When a person is healthy, his bio-energies are in balance. In such a state, they perform and control all physiological functions and are called *dhatu* (substances that support the body). If the balance is disturbed, all physiological functions are scrambled, which means the onset of illness. Such a diminished state is called *dosha* (disturbance). If the three bio-energies are out of balance for a prolonged period of time or are severely disturbed, they become toxic and must be removed from the body. They are then called *mala* (substances that must be removed from the body).

However, bio-energies can never be completely eliminated from the body (just waste products can) nor can they be converted into body tissue.

The three bio-energies have developed from the five elements. Thus, the dominant element determines the character of the respective bio-energy. *Vata* is a combination of the elements ether and air. The dominant element in *pitta* is fire, with the element water playing a minor role, because the so-called fire of digestion is not an open fire in the stomach and the small intestines in the literal sense, but rather the presence of enzymatic digestive juices. *Kapha* is a combination of the elements water and earth.

The relatively narrow range of balance of the three bio-energies assures that all psychosomatic activities in the body function perfectly. This represents ayurvedic health. Even a small deviation from the norm of one or more bio-energies is a sign of a diseased state in which the three bio-energies are hyperactive or hypoactive. Ayurvedic medicine does not wait until a person shows symptoms of an illness that, in the worst scenario, either cannot be cured at all or requires very powerful medication. Instead, it acts when the cause of an illness manifests itself. Ayurvedic science talks about minimal, distinctive, or extreme hypoactivity or hyperactivity of one or more bio-energies. In cases of hyperactivity, ayurvedic medicine uses antagonistic measures (substances with opposing characteristics); in cases of hypoactivity, it uses measures or substances that are similar in their characteristics.

Basic Elements of Bio-Energies

Elements	Bio-Energies	Characteristics of the Bio-Energies
Ether } Air }	*Vata*	Dry, cold, mobile, light, penetrating, clear, rough
Fire	*Pitta*	Slightly oily, hot, mobile, liquid, penetrating, sour, sharp
Water } Earth }	*Kapha*	Oily, cold, immobile, heavy, soft, sweet, mucous

For example, many rheumatic illnesses can be traced to a hyperactive *vata*. Heat is an antagonistic measure, which means that the rheumatic symptoms can be relieved with heat therapy. Patients afflicted with rheumatism can be found in every spa, where symptoms usually are lessened because of the temperature of the water. Similarly, a cold glass of water quenches thirst, which means it reduces *pitta* and *vata*, but increases *kapha*. The opposite result is achieved when the water is heated; it warms the body, increases *pitta*, and reduces *kapha* and *vata*.

Vata won't show any physical signs, but it can be observed by watching the different processes it sets in motion.

Pitta and *kapha* have a fluid character; *pitta* is lighter, and *kapha* is heavier.

30

Bio-Energy *Vata*

Vata has the characteristics of the elements ether and air; so, it is dry, light, subtle, coarse, unsteady, and clear. Substances with antagonistic characteristics normalize hyperactivity and weaken hypoactivity. Although all three bio-energies are important, *vata* is special. There is no bodily function that is not guided by *vata,* because *pitta* and *kapha* are considered slow or sluggish. Motion-inducing power is missing in both. For this reason, *vata* plays a significant role in every therapy. Only *vata* can expel toxic substances from the body, dry out wounds, and stimulate healing in diseased organs.

Vata controls cell division; the formation of cell layers; the differentiation of organs; and the activities of the heart, lung, stomach, and intestines. It also guides the impulses the brain and spine receive from the senses; initiates the activities of the tactile organs (the motor organs); evacuates waste material, such as stool, urine, perspiration, menstruation, semen, and the fetus. *Vata* is the driving force of all human activity.

Professor M. M. Shastry describes the movement of *vata* (not unlike the formula of Ohm's law) as being in direct proportion to its power of motivation and the resistance in the body's channels (and tissues). Thus,

$$\frac{vata's \text{ motivational power}}{\text{resistance of channels}} = vata's \text{ motion}$$

All three bio-energies exist throughout the body. In general, however, we can say that *kapha* resides in the upper part of the body, *pitta* in the middle part, and *vata* in the lower part. However, Caraka also lists specific parts of the body where normal *vata* bio-energies are located. These are the bladder, rectum, pelvis, upper thighs, feet, bones, and lower intestines. Other authors, such as Vagbhata, add the skin, ears, and nervous system. In addition, all three bio-energies are divided into five subgroups.

Pranavata   *Prana* means "life's air." *Pranavata* supports the vital functions of respiration, heart rate, and other vegetative functions, such as swallowing, spitting, sneezing, and burping. In addition, *pranavata* supports mental, intellectual, and sensory abilities, and, therefore, aids concentration. When *pranavata* is out of balance, it is possible for a person to experience sensory disturbances in specific parts of the body, as hypersensitivity, or even mental confusion. In general, *pranavata* is responsible for our ability to experience the presence of air, water, food, and sensory stimuli. This process moves from the outside to the inside.

Udanavata Here, the process moves in exactly the opposite direction—from the inside to the outside. *Udanavata* includes verbal expression, enthusiasm, vitality, strength, physical and psychic efforts, face and body color, and more.

To remember means to recall facts, bringing the internal to the "outside." This knowledge was originally stored through the power of *pranavata*. Thus, remembering ("knowing") also belongs to *udanavata*. Any disturbance can lead to the loss of energy and zest for life.

Vyanavata *Vyanavata* is the driving force that moves from the center to the periphery. It guides automatic movements, transports nutrients via the heart and circulatory system, and causes perspiration. As described by Susruta, it guides five different types of movement (expansion, contraction, and the movement of energy from the center in upward, downward, and lateral directions). Problems in the circulatory system and a general slowing of the body are part of *vyanavata*.

Samanavata The main functions of the *samanavata* (which lies in the vicinity of the digestive energy, *pacakapitta*) are the neural control of the secretion of the different digestive juices, the movements within the digestive channels, the separation of nutrients and waste products, and the transport of those nutrients. When disturbed, an insufficient amount of stomach juices are produced, causing loss of appetite, loss of weight, and the like.

Apanavata The word *apana* means "the lower end" and describes the lower portion of the spinal cord. *Apanavata* separates fluids from solid material in the colon. It guides the process of urination, the erection of the penis, the ejaculation of semen, the flow of menstruation, and the contractions of the uterus during the birthing process. Disturbances can cause infertility, impotence, miscarriages, constipation, flatulence, and so forth.

A careful study of the five subgroups of *vata* shows that a few functions of *vata* have not yet been discussed—emotions, maintaining a balance between body and spirit, the formation of the seven body tissues, and cell division.

Hypoactivity of *vata* is similar to a hyperactive *kapha,* resulting in a sensation of heaviness in the body, sluggishness, and insufficient blood circulation.

Hyperactivity of *vata* leads to dehydration; rough, dark, discolored skin; paralysis; increased stool; a feeling of coldness; poorly healing wounds; and premature aging.

Hyperactivity of *Vata* Occurs

In the early morning hours—around 4 A.M.
In the late afternoon—about 4 P.M.
After the age of 60
After the process of digestion is completed
After the intake of food that is light, dry, very cold, or small in quantity
When the weather is cold and dry
After intense athletic activity
After overexertion
After intercourse
After an injury
After a cold bath
When exhausted
When losing body tissue
When grieving
During anxiety attacks
When worrying
During intense moments of joy
After being frightened
During periods of insomnia

Bio-Energy *Pitta*

The bio-energy *pitta* consists of the element fire and a small portion of the element water. One might ask how two such contrary elements can be combined. The element fire is much more than an open flame. Burning can also be caused by fluids through enzymatic activities and by acids.

The characteristics of *pitta* are sharp, sour, hot, liquid, slightly oily, penetrating, and mobile. This energy has the smell of raw flesh. Substances with similar characteristics will increase *pitta*; those with opposite characteristics will reduce *pitta*. Susruta wrote that a weakened *pitta* energy can be healed with medication and therapies that create warmth; while a hypoactive *pitta* can be healed with medication and therapy that have cooling effects—just as one would handle a real fire.

Pitta produces body tissues (*dhatu*), waste products (*mala*), and bio-energies (*dosha*) from food. *Pitta* guides metabolism, is responsible for all gastrointestinal secretions (stomach and intestines), and controls body temperatures, hunger, thirst, discoloration of the skin, suppleness, and the ability to see. In the psychological arena, *pitta* deals with courage, intellect, clarity, bravery, and cheerfulness. Although *pitta* is present in every part of the body, it resides mainly between the navel and the nipples. It can also be found in the sweat glands, lymph nodes, stomach, and the small intestine. There are five subgroups.

Pacakapitta   *Pacakapitta* is responsible for the primary breakdown of food. *Samanavata* stimulates its secretion. The prominent place that *pacakapitta* occupies is mentioned in every textbook. All other functions of *pitta* depend on the condition of *pacakapitta*. A diminished function leads not only to problems in the digestive system, but also plays a role in other illnesses.

Ranjakapitta   The production of blood (*rakta*) and plasma (*rasa*) is controlled by *ranjakapitta*, which also plays a secondary role in the digestive process. It is located in the liver and the spleen. A disturbance leads to a deficiency in hemoglobin.

Sadhakapitta   References in classical texts suggest that *sadhakapitta* is closely related to higher mental abilities and can, therefore, be considered to have a psychophysiological function. This, in turn, is closely related to the metabolism of the nervous system and the synthesis of neurohormonal substances. The rapid process of relaying and converting sensory stimuli is also governed by this energy. Disturbances lead to mental sluggishness, deficient intelligence, and to feelings of hopelessness.

Alocakapitta   The natural function of *pitta* is conversion. The function of *alocakapitta* in the *drishti mandala* (retina) of the eye is the conversion of light rays (energies of the visible spectrum) into potential action of the optical nerve (*vata*). A disturbance of *alocakapitta* results in a diminished ability to see.

Bhrajakapitta   The production of normal or discolored skin, the aura of the body, the absorption and conversion of substances applied to the skin, and the control of the body's temperature depend on *bhrajakapitta*. All these activities are the result of metabolism and are closely related to the nutrition the body receives. Disturbances of *bhrajakapitta* cause different discolorations of the skin and poor complexion. In addition, body temperature is out of control, and the skin loses its ability to absorb.

Hypoactivity of *pitta* usually creates constipation, sensitivity to cold, and a pale complexion. The symptoms are similar to those caused by hyperactivity of *vata* and *kapha*.

Hyperactivity of *pitta* gives skin, urine, and stool a yellowish color. It leads to extreme sensations of hunger and thirst; a craving for something cold; a burning sensation of the skin, hands, and eyes; hypersensitivity; allergies; eczema; dizziness; fever; and psychological disturbances, such as anger, hate, and jealousy. This hyperactivity can also lead to infectious diseases.

Hyperactivity of *Pitta* Occurs
At noon
Around midnight
In middle age
During digestion
After consuming food that is hot, salty, sour, or very spicy
During a fast
When hunger and thirst are ignored
During exposure to strong sunlight
During hot weather
When feeling angry and hateful
During intensive intellectual activities

Bio-Energy *Kapha*

The third bio-energy is *kapha*. It consists of the elements water and earth. These elements take care of the structural integrity of the body. The characteristics are heavy, cold, soft, stable, mucous, and sweet. Hyperactivity should be complemented with substances that have opposite characteristics. During hypoactivity, look for substances that have the same characteristics.

Kapha is responsible for lubrication, for holding the skeletal structure together (particularly the joints), and for supporting stability and weight. In addition, it is responsible for sexual potency and fertility and for resistance to illnesses and deterioration. Also included are emotional capacities, such as patience, inner strength, and lack of desire. The enormous heat produced by *pitta* must be balanced by *kapha*. At the same time, body tissues must be protected from stress and the wear and tear created by *vata*. In addition, appropriate fluids ensure that the products of the biochemical processes are properly distributed throughout the body. In this sense, *kapha* takes care of homeostasis.

The upper parts of the body are considered the seat of *kapha;* however, it can also be found in other parts of the body. The upper chest is considered to be the special place where *kapha* resides. In addition, the head, neck, throat, joints, upper abdomen, and fatty tissues are mentioned as probable locations of this energy. There are five subgroups of *kapha*.

Avalambakakapha Much wear and tear takes place during the constant contraction and expansion of the lungs, heart muscle, and central part of the intestines. Useful protection is provided through very minute secretions of fluids controlled by *avalambakakapha*. Disturbances lead to increased heartbeat and to heart and lung weaknesses.

Kledakakapha   This energy ensures that the stomach and other internal organs are not "digested" by the strong digestive juices (*pitta*). In addition, it also protects these organs from foods that are too hot or too cold. The mucus in the stomach is able to do this by moistening the food and breaking it down into molecules. Gastritis and ulcers in the small intestine are often the result of weak mucous membranes.

Tarpakakapha   Susruta writes that this energy is located in the brain. Its purpose is to maintain strength and to keep brain tissues moist and cool. The modern term for this is *cerebrospinal fluid.*

Bodhakakapha   *Bodhakakapha* gives a person the ability to taste. Dangerous substances usually taste very bad and can be immediately spat out. Taste receptors react only to substances that are dissolved in the fluids present in the oral cavity. Saliva aids speaking, is the first stage of the digestive process, and has antibacterial properties. Losing the sense of taste is a sign of a disturbed *bodhakakapha*.

Sleshakakapha   The main functions of this energy are to keep all joints in the body well moistened and to protect tissue surfaces in contact with each other. Weakness and premature wear of joints are signs of a disturbed *sleshakakapha*.

Hypoactivity of *kapha* usually leads to a sense of hollowness, increased heart rate, and to joints that feel "loose." The stability and resistance of the tissues are reduced, and the mind and emotions become vulnerable. These symptoms are similar to those of a hyperactive *vata*.

Hyperactivity of *kapha* leads to a loss of appetite, nausea, vomiting, sense of heaviness, swollen joints, cough accompanied by heavy phlegm, excessive need for sleep, lethargy, loss of concentration, and lack of blood.

Hyperactivity of *Kapha* Occurs
In the morning—around 8 A.M.
In the evening—around 8 P.M.
Immediately after a meal
After a meal consisting of sweet, oily, fatty, and cold food, as well as
   watery fruits and vegetables, such as melons, cucumbers, oranges, and
   grapes

After excessive water intake
When physically inactive
During cold and wet weather
When greedy, miserly, and attached to material possessions

The Seven Body Tissues (*Sapta Dhatu*)

The basic tissues that make up and support the body are called *dhatu*. During normal states (except during reproduction) these tissues are never eliminated from the body. The body cannot afford to lose any of these vital substances. If loss does occur, serious illnesses result.

During the process of metabolism, tissues are separated from waste products. So-called digested food, the fundamental base of *sapta dhatu*, undergoes seven consecutive evolutionary stages, during which the potential energy of each increases. (See table, The Seven Body Tissues.)

The Seven Body Tissues

Tissue	Type	Function
Plasma (*rasa*)	Circulating nutrients	Nutrition
Blood (*rakta*)	Hemoglobin portion of the blood	Oxygen exchange
Muscle (*mamsa*)	Muscle tissue	Movement
Fat (*meda*)	Fat tissue	Lubrication
Bones (*asthi*)	Bone tissue	Support
Nerves (*majja*)	Bone marrow and nerve tissue	Flow of information
Semen (*shukra*)	Reproductive tissue	Reproduction

While bio-energies are the cause of illnesses, body tissues are the place where illnesses manifest themselves. In general, *kapha* energy is responsible for all body tissues, particularly plasma, muscle, fat, bone, and the tissues of the ovum and semen. Disturbances in any of these tissues weakens the tissues that develop subsequently. In the course of development, each tissue undergoes different changes. Due to the effects of the digestive capacity of each tissue (*agni*), stable, or solid, parts (*sthayi*) develop. In the course of this digestive process, secondary tissues (*upadhatu*) are formed and tissue-specific waste products (*mala*) are produced. The result of this cleansing process produces formative tissues (*asthayi*), which are the basic product for the tissues that develop next.

Weak tissue metabolism leads to the formation of too much tissue, which is also of poor quality. If metabolism increases, too little tissue is formed; instead, it literally burns. The more defined, specific types of tissues (as well as those that are more general in nature) are used to store energy. For instance, blood is concentrated plasma, muscle tissue is concentrated blood, and fat tissue is concentrated muscle tissue. While plasma is formed everyday by food intake, the formation of the other *dhatu* involves a longer, more drawn-out process. For instance, it takes about 35 days for reproductive tissue to form from plasma. Reproductive

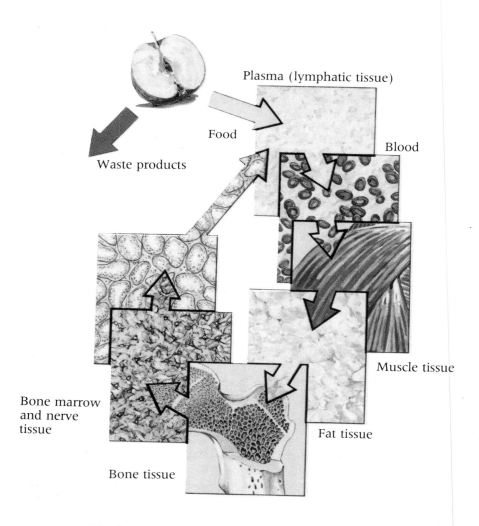

The formation of body tissue (*sapta dhatu*) from food

tissue supports all other tissue, just as every tissue supports those that are developing next, closing the circle.

Plasma

Rasa dhatu is the fundamental substance of the body and is most easily compared to lymph. This protein-containing liquid circulates throughout the body and supplies nutrition to all types of tissues. Plasma provides fluids for the body and maintains the equilibrium of the electrolytes. Plasma is present throughout the body, but it resides mainly in the heart, blood vessels, lymph system, skin, and soft body tissues.

If *rasa dhatu* is present in sufficient amounts, the result is vitality, the urge for movement and activity, and a sense of beauty and joy. The word *rasa* can be translated as "joy of life" or "essence of life."

* When too little of this basic substance is present, the skin and lips become rough and dry. Other symptoms are tiredness, sensitivity to noise, jittery muscles, increased pulse, and a sense of emptiness in the heart.

* When present in excess, there is an increase of mucus and saliva, channels in the body are blocked, dizziness and lack of appetite set in, and *kapha* increases throughout the body.

The secondary tissues of plasma are milk and menstrual flow. *Kapha* produces plasma and its waste products.

Blood

Red blood cells provide needed oxygen to the blood. Sufficient oxygen creates a healthy body and skin color. Many illnesses result from oxygen deficiency in the tissues. A person with a sufficient amount of blood radiates energy and possesses love and trust.

* Deficiencies cause pale skin, low blood pressure, shock, craving for sour and cold foods, a sense of dryness in the head, loss of radiance, and dry and cracked skin.

* Too much *rakta dhatu* leads to skin diseases, abscesses, enlargement of the liver and spleen, high blood pressure, ulcers, hepatitis, delirium, burning sensations, and reddening of the skin, eyes, and urine.

The secondary tissues (*upadhatu*) of the blood form blood vessels and tendons. The waste product (*mala*) is *pitta*, which produces *dhatu*. However, if there is too much blood tissue present, it also turns into a waste product, leading to hyperactivity of *pitta*.

Muscle Tissue

Muscle tissue makes motion and movements possible and holds the body together. If this tissue is well developed, the body has strength, self-confidence, and courage.

- Deficiencies lead to thinness or emaciation, particularly in the hip area, belly, and neck. Tiredness develops, limbs become weak, and co-ordination decreases. Insecurity is the result.

- Overproduction of *mamsa dhatu* leads to swelling or tumors of the muscle tissues, swelling of the lymph nodes, obesity, enlargement of the liver, irritability, and aggression. In women, it can lead to fibrous tissue in the uterus, which can result in miscarriages and infertility.

Ligaments and skin are secondary muscle tissues. Discharges from the navel, outer ear, and ear wax are some of the waste products.

Fatty Tissue

Fat is responsible for keeping muscles, ligaments, and joints lubricated. It provides a person with a good voice. Psychologically, it gives a sense of being cared for, which is why many people gain weight trying to coun-teract a sense that they are not lovable.

- Too little *meda dhatu* leads to weakness, cracking joints, tiredness, tired eyes, enlargement of the spleen, emaciation, and brittle hair, nails, bones, and teeth.

- Too much leads to obesity, tiredness, lack of movement, asthma, sexual weakness, thirst, high blood pressure, and a fat belly. Emotionally, it leads to an obsession with material things and to fear.

Abdominal fat is the secondary tissue formed from fat tissue. The waste product is sweat.

Bone Tissue

Asthi dhatu supports all body tissues. That also holds true for a person's psychological state. Healthy bone tissue ensures security, stability, and endurance. *Vata* is located in the bone tissue.

- Deficiencies result in extreme tiredness, painful and weak joints, loss of teeth and hair, and brittle nails.

- Excessive bone tissue causes bone deformations, spurs, extra teeth, an overly large physique, painful joints, lack of endurance, arthritis, and cancer of the bone.

Secondary tissues form teeth; waste products are hair and nails.

Bone Marrow and Nerve Tissue

One of the functions of bone marrow is to fill the hollow spaces of the body. It also produces joint fluids and fluids to moisten the eyes, skin, and stool. When it is present in sufficient quantity, bone marrow gives a feeling of fulfillment. If it is not, a feeling of emptiness and anxiety results.

• Too little bone marrow can cause weakening and porosity of the bones, painful joints, dizziness, dark circles under the eyes, sexual weakness, a feeling of emptiness, and anxieties. *Vata* diseases often lead to a deficit of nerve tissue.

• Too much *majja dhatu* causes a feeling of heaviness in the limbs, dulling and infections of the eyes, and makes wounds difficult to heal.

The secondary tissue of bone marrow and nerve tissue is the fluid in the eye socket; tears and secretions of the eyes are the waste products.

Reproductive Tissue

The role of reproductive tissue is to create new life. *Shukra* literally means "semen," but it also refers to ovum and generative fluids in general.

• A deficit in reproductive tissue leads to a lack of strength, a lack of or slow ejaculation, impotence, weak immune responses, back pain in the lumbar region, dry mucous membranes, insecurity, and an absence of libido.

• Too much *shukra dhatu* leads to extreme sexual drives and fits of anger. It can also cause the development of stones in semen fluid and an enlarged prostate.

Secondary reproductive tissue is called *ojas,* the subtle essence of all body tissue. Its waste product is smegma.

Shukra dhatu maintains the functioning of the autoimmune system. Proper immune protection is only guaranteed if a sufficient amount of *shukra dhatu* is present. Extreme sexual activity diminishes *shukra dhatu.* According to ayurveda, it is no accident that the AIDS virus is spreading fast among people who are extremely sexually active (heterosexually, bisexually, or homosexually) and among those whose body tissue is systematically destroyed by the use of drugs.

Reproductive tissue is only formed after all other *dhatu* tissue has sufficiently developed and matured. This means that it is very important to ensure that all other tissues have a chance to fully and properly develop during early childhood and prepubescence. It is said that the extreme sexual stimulation that youth is exposed to leads to premature development of *shukra dhatu*. If children or young people are already exposed to sexual activity, permanent damage to bone, nerve, and other tissues results.

Some authors have called *ojas* the eighth tissue, representing the essence of all other tissues, but having no physical substance itself. They have named it the "juices of life's energy." It is located near the heart chakra.

We have focused on the seven body tissues. As we have already mentioned, the potential of subsequent tissue is always higher than the one preceding it. Plasma becomes blood, blood becomes muscle tissue, muscle tissue becomes fat tissue, fat tissue becomes bone tissue, bone tissue becomes bone marrow, bone marrow becomes reproductive tissue. The last tissue, *shukra dhatu*, is the one with the highest potential.

Bodily Waste Product (*Mala*)

Mala is the substance that is constantly eliminated from the body. This includes material such as stool, urine, and sweat. Waste products react correspondingly to hypoactivity or hyperactivity of the three bio-energies and seven body tissues. The different characteristics are described in more detail in the Pathology and Diagnoses chapter. Waste products with much finer structures (*sukshma mala* or *kleda*) leave the body through pores in the epithelium, the uppermost layer of the skin, and through the mucous membranes. In addition, we have described *dhatu mala*, which is a product of the process of potentialization of tissues.

A healthy state can only be achieved if waste products are eliminated early enough. Accumulation of waste products automatically leads to disturbance of bio-energies and, in turn, to illnesses.

Bio-Typology
Prakriti Pariksha

Ayurveda does not consider illness an isolated occurrence; illness is always discussed in connection with the individual's constitution. On one hand, we have a disturbance of the bio-energies *vata, pitta,* and *kapha;* and on the other hand, we have a unique person. In addition to different physical and psychological characteristics, human beings can also be categorized according to the dominance of one of the bio-energies.

In addition to ur-matter, *prakriti* has another meaning. In connection with the topic discussed here, it means "the constitutional basis of an individual," in short, "bio-type." This bio-type, or *prakitri,* is determined at the time of conception and is influenced by many different factors. The hereditary qualities of semen and ovum play the most prominent role. In addition, the nutrition of the expectant mother, prevailing bio-energetic conditions, psyche, consciousness, location, and constellation all play a part; however, these are secondary factors.

Caraka and other authors distinguish between four bio-types.

> **Vata prakriti**—a person with a dominant *vata* bio-energy
> **Pitta prakriti**—a person with a dominant *pitta* bio-energy
> **Kapha prakriti**—a person with a dominant *kapha* bio-energy
> **Sama prakriti**—a person with balanced bio-energies

Of course, in real life we always deal with combinations of bio-energies, which is why we use the terms *dominant* or *prominent.* Other authors, such as Vagbhata, also talk about combinations of two bio-types. However, for the sake of simplicity, we prefer the use of four subdivisions.

The characteristics of the dominant bio-energy also determine the character of the person. Thus, every person reacts differently to different environmental influences, misfortunes, nutrition, medications, and physical therapies. Neither "assembly-line" medical treatment nor mass-produced medication can guarantee improvements or healing. The same holds true for catchy phrases, such as "fasting is good for everybody." Every ayurvedic treatment is based on the principle of bio-type, and no person is treated until his or her bio-type has been established.

In earlier times, physicians and pharmacists prepared medications for each patient individually, often with pestle and mortar. They usually knew the prominent characteristics of their clients, and they took those into consideration in deciding therapies. However, they had to work without the benefit of a scientific theory, such as ayurveda. For that reason, they had nothing to counter the arguments of modern scientists. Today, this situation has totally changed, because dissatisfied and better-informed consumers do not accept standardized therapies or standard medications. They are looking for alternatives. A prevailing opinion is that modern scientists were unable to keep their promises.

Determining Bio-Types

With the help of the following test, you will be able to determine your own individual constitution. Armed with that information, you will find the corresponding diet plan in the Nutritional Science chapter and life-confirming measures in the Life-Style chapter that follows. Both will surely help improve the quality of your life.

Every human being has a right to a long, healthy life. Everyone should actively fight for this right. About three and a half centuries ago, Caraka stated, "In general, human activities revolve around religion, economic improvement, the pursuit of happiness, and spiritual emancipation. All these goals can only be achieved as long as we possess a healthy mind and a healthy body. Therefore, the most important human activity is the protection and preservation of health." Hard work, ambitions, and the strictest adherence to moral standards are for naught once we are dead. Think of the effort necessary to save for a car or a house, often at the expense of our health. Illnesses and death, however, are not just statistical data insurance companies use. They can be directly influenced by every person. Prevention of illnesses should be our greatest concern.

The following **Bio-Type Test** consists of a number of characteristics and symptoms that are directly connected to the three bio-energies. Read every question carefully and mark the appropriate box. When in doubt, choose the answer closest to what you think it should be. After you have answered all questions, add the boxes you have marked in each column. Give each answer one point.

If column 1 has the highest number of points, you are a vata *person. The highest number of points in column 2 indicates a* pitta *type. The highest number of points in column 3 identifies you as a* kapha *type.*

44

Bio-Type Test

	Vata		Pitta		Kapha	
Do you tend to be	Underweight	☐	Ideal with good muscles	☐	Overweight	☐
Is your frame	Small boned	☐	Normal	☐	Large boned	☐
Are you	Very short	☐	Medium height	☐	Small and stout	☐
	Very tall	☐			Large and stout	☐
Are your hips	Narrow	☐	Medium	☐	Wide	☐
Are your shoulders	Narrow	☐	Medium	☐	Wide	☐
Is your chest	Flat	☐	Normally developed	☐	Fully developed	☐
Is your hair	Normal	☐	Balding, prematurely grey	☐	Full	☐
Has your face	Irregular features	☐	Prominent features	☐	Round features	☐
Are your eyes	Small	☐	Medium	☐	Large	☐
	Dry	☐	Red	☐	Moist	☐
Is your nose	Small	☐	Medium	☐	Large	☐
	Small, long	☐	Straight, pointed	☐	Wide	☐
Are your lips	Small, rather dark	☐	Medium, red, soft	☐	Wide, velvety	☐
Are your teeth	Not straight	☐	Medium, straight	☐	Large, straight	☐
Are you fingers	Small, long	☐	Regular	☐	Wide, angular	☐
Are your nails	Brittle	☐	Soft	☐	Strong, thick	☐
Are your feet	Small, narrow	☐	Medium	☐	Large, wide	☐
Are your hands and feet	Cold, dry	☐	Warm, pink	☐	Cool, damp	☐
Is your skin	Dry	☐	Freckled	☐	Soft and smooth	☐
	Brownish	☐	Radiant	☐	Light, white	☐
Are your veins	Easily visible	☐	Evenly distributed	☐	Not visible	☐
Where is your fat	Around the waist	☐	Evenly distributed	☐	Around thighs and buttocks	☐
Are you	Hyperactive	☐	Active	☐	Somewhat lethargic	☐
Do you walk	Rather fast	☐	Normally	☐	Rather slowly	☐
Is your sleep	Light and interrupted	☐	Short and even	☐	Long and deep	☐
Is your thirst	Variable	☐	Good	☐	Not noticeable	☐

	Vata		Pitta		Kapha	
Is your appetite	Variable	☐	Strong	☐	Moderate	☐
Is your perspiration	Sparse, odorless	☐	Heavy with a strong odor	☐	Heavy with a pleasant odor	☐
Is the amount of your urine	Little, but frequent	☐	Normal, but often	☐	Profuse, infrequent	☐
Is your stool	Hard, dark Constipation	☐	Loose, yellowish Diarrhea	☐	Soft, well formed	☐
					Normal	☐
Is your creativity	Distinct and rich in ideas	☐	Inventive and technical or scientific	☐	In the area of business	☐
Is your memory	Average	☐	Excellent	☐	Good	☐
Is your decision-making ability	Problematic	☐	Quick, decisive	☐	Well thought out	☐
Is your speech	Fast	☐	Loud	☐	Melodic	☐
When handling money, are you	Wasteful	☐	Methodical	☐	Thrifty	☐
Are you	Shy	☐	Jealous	☐	Solicitous	☐
	Nervous	☐	Ambitious	☐	Lethargic	☐
	Insecure	☐	Egotistical	☐	Self-satisfied	☐
	Intuitive	☐	Practical	☐	Resilient	☐
Is your sexual drive	Extreme or the opposite	☐	Passionate and domineering	☐	Constant and loyal	☐
Do you love	Travel	☐	Sports	☐	Quiet	☐
	Art	☐	Politics	☐	Business	☐
	Esoteric subjects	☐	Luxury	☐	Good food	☐
Do you dislike	Cold, wind, and dryness	☐	Heat and midday sun	☐	Cold and dampness	☐
Evaluation	*Vata* **Total**	☐	*Pitta* **Total**	☐	*Kapha* **Total**	☐

The *Vata* Person

People with low body weight and a light bone structure belong to the *vata* type. A typical characteristic is a prominent Adam's apple. This type is very enthusiastic, fast to act, and tends to be forgetful. Sometimes this person talks more than he should. His creativity is in the artistic domain. He loves esoteric material, is able to detect clairvoyant or healing powers within himself, and lives an ascetic life-style. By nature, he is shy and sensitive. It may be he quits school early and changes jobs often.

Since the bio-energy *vata* is dominant, this person is very prone to all *vata* illnesses. These are rheumatism, nervous disorders, sciatica, insomnia, dry skin, constipation, receding gums, weak bones, infertility, impotence, a weak heart, colic, flatulence, stuttering, ringing in the ears, irregular menstruation with cramps, varicose veins, paralysis, blood clotting, anorexia, shivering fits, poor blood circulation, and more.

Vata types need jobs that do not consist of extreme physical activities. Their workplace should be in a warm and protected location. In addition, they should not have to work where constant concentration is required, otherwise, their health may be strongly impaired.

The *Pitta* Person

The *pitta* person holds the middle ground between the *vata* and *kapha* person. Thanks to his well-functioning metabolism and urge for physical activity, he has a healthy body with well-developed muscles. This type is always alert. His ambition allows him to go far in life. His creativity is methodical, inventive, and usually connected to technical or scientific subjects. He is a good speaker and sells himself and his products well. Aggressiveness can change into hostility and impatience. His hair will turn grey sooner than is the case with other types, and there is a tendency towards baldness. He must have sufficient food and drink and must eat and drink regularly. His mental abilities are good; he has an excellent memory, and he loves intellectual activities.

Constant stress and too much excitement often lead to high blood pressure. He is prone to coronary diseases (thrombosis). Other dangers include stomach ulcers; tumors; stomach, intestinal, and skin cancer; psoriasis; inflammation of the lymph system; infectious diseases; inflammation of the spleen; hepatitis; infections of the urinary tract; heartburn; herpes; very heavy menstruation; and similar illnesses.

This bio-type must be challenged in his work. His workplace should not be near a heat source.

The *Kapha* Person

People with a heavy, solid body structure belong to the *kapha* type. They possess strength and endurance. Although they take their time when attending to their work, they are secure and self-confident, which usually allows them to achieve prosperity.

They are not easily rattled and are sometimes lethargic. They love to let others work for them, which they usually pull off rather well, because they have an excellent entrepreneurial sense. Their positive side is reliability, patience, politeness, and generosity. Their negative side is distinct materialism, greed, passivity, and a tendency to sleep too much and too often.

People from this group often tend to be overweight, have a lack of appetite, a weak digestive system, insufficient circulation, vomiting, flu, colds, bronchitis, asthma, kidney stones, swollen lymph nodes, benign tumors, dropsy, goiter, lung and breast cancer, fungal infections, and similar illnesses.

This body type is good for heavy physical work. Extreme sedentary living tends to result in weight gain. The *kapha* person is well suited for public service, entrepreneurial activities, and a leadership position in a company. If the place where he works is not protected from dampness, he will suffer from joint pain.

The Balanced Person

From a physical, emotional, and psychological point of view, this is the ideal type. All three bio-energies are well balanced. This bio-type suffers less often from emotional ups and downs and is also well protected from illnesses. If he should get sick, it is usually caused by poor nutrition or by external (climate, time of year, etc.) influences. Well-balanced people take note of even the smallest details. They follow a very well designed daily routine, because they believe that success never comes easily.

They are considered important models and often hold very important positions in society. Sadly, they are very rare.

Of course, there is always the possibility of having an equal amount of points in two categories. Such types have the qualities of those two bio-types.

Anatomical Aspects
Sharira

Srotas (Body Channels)

The human body consists of a huge system of different channels (*srotas*) that supply nutrition to tissues and organs and contribute to the task of keeping the whole organism clean. These channels have a certain physical structure and very specific functions (*Caraka Samhita*, Nidana Sthana). Caraka, however, dismissed the notion that the human body is only the sum of these channels. He argued that *srotas* only provide circulation and are to be defined by the substances they carry and their destinations.

Srotas are networks of "open spaces" in the body. An undisturbed flow through these channels indicates health. Illness, on the other hand, can develop when any of four different malfunctions occurs.

Excessive Circulation This takes place when too many substances are transported through the channels, or when these substances are moving too fast. Excessive circulation creates hyperactivity, which can lead to overdevelopment of certain tissues and organs.

Inefficient Circulation This occurs when too few substances are moving through the channels or if they are moving too slowly, leading to hypoactivity. The result is an underdevelopment and dehydration of tissues or organs. In addition, waste products are not properly eliminated and are stored in the body.

Blocked Circulation A blockage occurs when bio-energies, bodily waste products, or undigested food (*ama*) accumulate and harden. This can lead to atrophy of whole organs and portions of tissues.

Damage to a Channel This is usually the result of a blockage. The circulating substances try to find a way around the blockage and come in direct contact with the surrounding tissues or organs. Since the substances are incompatible (they do not "fit" organically) with the tissues that they invade, considerable damage can result.

49

Excess bio-energies, waste products, and undigested food almost always lead to a disturbance in the circulatory channels. *Vata* plays the main role in the flow of the channels. These circulatory channels are somewhat similar to the different physiological systems of modern medicine; however, according to ayurvedic philosophy, they are also very similar to the meridian in Chinese medicine. Illnesses are classified according to the system that is involved.

Ayurvedic medicine has a complex symptomatology of the circulatory channels. Knowledge and the ability to diagnose the symptoms of an illness are very important tools in determining the nature, location, and state of an illness.

The body consists of several circulatory channels. Some transport the basic substance of body tissue (*dhatu*) to the next stage; others carry health-supporting or illness-carrying bio-energies; others eliminate waste products. Susruta describes the nine channels that have openings to the outside—eyes, ears, mouth, nose, anus, and urethra. Women have three additional openings—both breasts, from which milk flows (*stanya vaha srota*), and the genetic passage, through which menstruation flows (*artava vaha srota*).

The *Caraka-Samhita* lists 13 different systems and their functionings (*Vimana-Sthana*).

Prana Vaha Srota

These channels provide the bloodstream with *prana*, the "breath of life," from the outside. Primarily, they are the breathing organs, but they also include the heart and the colon. Their balance can be disrupted when natural bodily urges are repressed or when too much fatty or oily food is eaten. A disturbance causes rapid breathing and breathing problems, such as painful respiration. These symptoms are treated the same way that bronchitis is.

Anna Vaha Srota

The responsibility of the gastrointestinal tract is to transport food. Disturbances are due to irregular meals, improper foods, and a weak digestion. The symptoms are colic, vomiting, poor digestion, abnormal thirst, disturbed vision, etc. Treatment is the same as for digestive problems.

Udaka Vaha Srota

These channels are responsible for transporting serum (fluids containing mostly protein—the portion of blood plasma that does not coagulate) and lymph (protein-containing fluids that have their own channel system and are very important for the fluid exchanges between tissues). They are located in the gums (*talu*), the soft tissue in the mouth, and the pancreas (*kloman*) and are mainly responsible for sugar metabolism. Disturbances result from hot weather, excessive alcohol consumption, dry food, lack of water, and digestive disturbance. Symptoms are a dryness in the mouth and throat and extreme thirst.

The circulatory systems transport the seven body tissues (*dhatu*).

Rasa Vaha Srota

Plasma (the liquid portion of the blood and the lymph) is carried in these channels. They are disturbed by oily, cold, and heavy food, and by worries and anxiety. Symptoms are swelling of various body parts, emaciation, and breathing difficulties. These problems are removed by fasting.

Rakta Vaha Srota

These channels allow blood to circulate. All blood tissue (starting with the very small capillaries), the liver, and the spleen are part of this network. Alcohol, hot weather, sunstroke, and pungent and oily foods cause disturbances. Symptoms are a burning sensation of the skin, reddening of the skin, fever, bleeding, reddening of the eyes, and more. Phlebotomy is the treatment of choice in these cases.

Mamsa Vaha Srota

These channels transport muscle fibre. They are located near tendons and muscle fibres that are close to skin tissue. Chewing food improperly, eating indigestible foods, and going to sleep immediately after a meal cause blockage of these channels. Symptoms are varicose veins, muscle atrophy, and swelling in different parts of the body. Symptoms are removed by surgical intervention or cauterization.

Medo Vaha Srota

These are channels that transport fat tissue. They are primarily located in the kidneys and the abdominal area. They are disturbed by lack of physical activity, sleeping during the day, alcohol, and fatty foods. Symptoms are excessive perspiration, oily skin, white gums, swelling of different parts of the body, and abnormal thirst. Treatment is a reducing diet.

Ashti Vaha Srota

These take care of bone tissue and are usually located in the pelvic area, the site in the body with the largest bones. Susruta does not mention these channels. Damage to them is caused by excessive sports or physical activities and excessive food intake, resulting in hyperactivity of *vata*. Symptoms include pain felt in the bones and teeth and pathological changes of the hair and nails. *Panchakarma* cleansing is the treatment of choice.

Majja Vaha Srota

These are the channels that primarily transport cerebrospinal fluids, the fluids of the brain and the bone marrow. They are found in bones and joints. The flow of these fluids is disturbed after an injury, by stressing the bone structure, and by eating indigestible foods. Symptoms are painful finger joints, dizziness, fainting spells, and deep abscesses at the joints of the fingers. Eating sweet and bitter-tasting foods is recommended.

Shukra Vaha Srota

Reproductive tissues, including semen and ovaries, are transported through these channels. They are damaged by inopportune, excessive, or repressed sexual urges. Symptoms are impotence, delayed ejaculation, and ejaculated semen mixed with blood. Treatment includes eating sweet and bitter-tasting foods and a cleansing treatment.

Sveda Vaha Srota

These transport sweat. They are primarily located in fat tissues and hair follicles. An overweight person tends to perspire excessively. These channels can be disrupted through excessive physical activity, hot weather, alternating hot and cold foods, and psychological stress. Symptoms are excessive or insufficient perspiration and burning sensations in the skin. The symptoms are treated in the same way as fever.

Purisha Vaha Srota

These eliminate stool from the body. The channels are located in the colon and rectum. Overindulgence in food and eating before the last meal has been properly digested cause malfunctions. Symptoms are constipation, flatulence, watery stools, foul-smelling stools, and discomfort during elimination. Treatment is the same as for diarrhea.

Mutra Vaha Srota

This is the channel that eliminates urine via the urethra. A disturbance results if a person ignores the urge to urinate and instead eats or continues intercourse. Symptoms include excessive or incomplete urination, diminished sensitivity in the genitals, and constipation. Treatment is the same as for urine retention.

Vital Points (*Marmas*)

The vital points (*marmas*) are very important parts of ayurvedic anatomy. An injury to one of these points (for instance, penetration by a weapon or through a serious fall or burn) will lead to permanent damage or even death. Knowledge of these vital points is of special importance in Asian martial arts and in surgery. On the one hand, injury to any of these points could render the enemy harmless; on the other hand, only a well-trained surgeon would be able to save a patient or an organ after such an injury. The vital points are where life energies are concentrated. Muscles, fat, bones, veins, arteries, tendons, and joints meet at these points. The channels are the primary seat of the activating air principle, *vagu;* of *soma* (cooling moon); the fire element, *tejas;* and the three omni-substances, *sattva, rajas,* and *tamas;* as well as the perceptions of the five senses.

Vital Points

Location	Arrangement	Effects of Injuries
22 on the upper extremities	41 in the blood vessels	19 cause instant death
22 on the lower extremities	11 in the muscle fibres	33 result in premature death
12 in the abdominal and chest region	27 in tendons and ligaments	3 result in death if a foreign body (arrow, knife, bullet) has been driven through them
14 in the back	20 in joints	44 result in disability
37 in the neck and the head	8 within the bone structure	8 cause severe pain

Very early on, it was known that these vital points and systems could be strengthened by massage. Here, too, the master of martial arts provided the lead. Classical martial art and its massage techniques are still performed in the south of India. This type of martial art was brought to China and Japan through Buddhism.

53

The combination of medicinal oils, acupressure, synchro-massage, and many other specific measures have led to the high art of ayurvedic massage. These techniques can be employed very effectively in cases of polio, psychic disturbances, such as psychosis, and also during rejuvenation and cleansing therapies.

The vital points and their respective locations are classified according to their body tissue and the effects injuries have on these vital points. Their size, measured with a finger held horizontally, *anguli*, is about ¾ inch (2 cm). This system of measuring is also used for determining their location. There are 107 vital points in the human body.

The Effect of Acupressure on Vital Points

Marma	Size in Finger Widths	No.	Location	Tissue	Effect of Injury	Effect of Acupressure
1. *Talahridaya*	½	4	Center of palm and sole of feet	Muscle	Early death	Stimulates lungs
2. *Kshipra*	½	4	Between thumb and index finger and first and second toe	Tendon	Early death	Stimulates heart
3. *Kurca*	4	4	2A above *kshipra* and base of thumb and toes	Tendon	Disability	Sole of feet stimulates *alo-chaka pitta*
4. *Kurcashira*	1	4	Below wrist and below ankle	Tendon	Pain	Control of muscle spasms
5. *Manibhanda*	2	2	Center of waist	Joint	Pain	Relieves stiffness
6. *Gulpha*	2	2	Ankle joint	Joint	Pain	Relieves stiffness
7. *Indravasti*	½	4	Middle of forearm and middle of lower leg	Muscle	Early death	Stimulates digestion and intestines

Marma	Size in Finger Widths	No.	Location	Tissue	Effect of Injury	Effect of Acupressure
8. Kurpara	3	2	Elbow	Joint	Disability	Stimulates heart and spleen
9. Janu	3	2	Knee	Joint	Disability	Stimulates heart and spleen
10. Ani	½	4	3A above, elbow, and knee	Tendon	Disability	Controls muscle tension
11. Urvi	1	4	Middle of upper arm and thigh	Blood vessel	Disability	Stimulates udaka vaha srota
12. Lohitaksha	½	4	Center of armpit and groin	Blood vessel	Disability	Controls blood supply of legs
13. Kashadhara	1	2	2A above lohitaksha of the armpit	Tendon	Disability	Controls muscle tension
14. Vitapa	1	2	2A below lohitaksha of the groin	Blood vessel	Disabling	Controls muscle tension of belly
15. Guda	4	1	Around anus	Muscle	Fatal	Stimulates 1st chakra, reproduction and urine systems
16. Vasti	4	1	Between pubic bone and navel	Ligament	Fatal	Stimulates kapha
17. Nabhi	4	1	Around navel	Ligament	Fatal	Stimulates small intestines and pacakapitta

Continued on p. 58

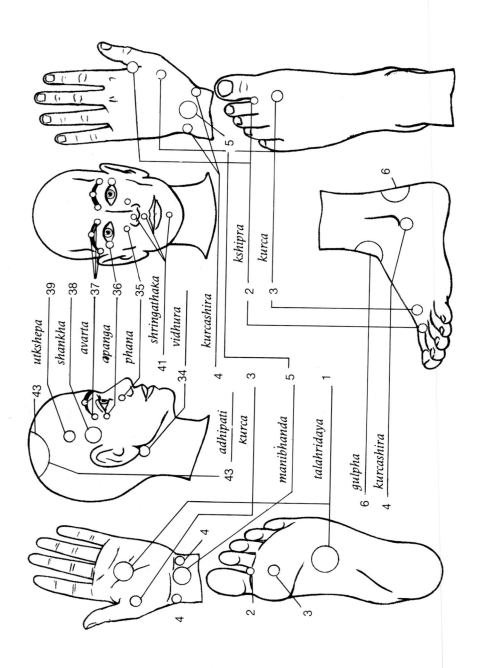

The Vital Points on the Hands, Feet, and Head

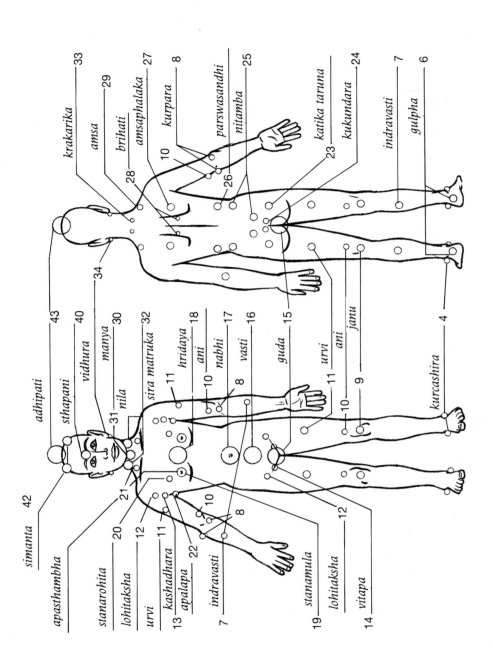

The Vital Points of the Body

57

Marma	Size in Finger Widths	No.	Location	Tissue	Effect of Injury	Effect of Acupressure
Continued from p. 55						
18. Hridaya	4	1	Center of breastbone	Blood vessel	Fatal	Stimulates sadhaka-pitta and vyana-vata
19. Stanamula	2	2	Below the nipples	Blood vessel	Premature death	Regulates blood circulation
20. Stanarohita	½	2	2A above stanamula	Muscle	Premature death	Relaxes arm muscles
21. Apasthambha	½	2	Center between nipples and collarbone	Blood vessel	Premature death	Influences sympathetic and parasympathetic nerves
22. Apalapa	½	2	Center of armpit, laterally from stanarohita	Blood vessel	Premature death	Influences sympathetic and parasympathetic nerves
23. Katika Taruna	½	2	Cheeks of buttocks, center of hips	Bone	Premature death	Stimulates fat tissue
24. Kukundara	½	2	Both sides of coccyx	Joint	Disability	Stimulates 2nd chakra
25. Nitamba	½	2	4A above and laterally from kukundara	Bone	Premature death	Stimulates production of red blood cells
26. Parswasandhi	½	2	2A above nitamba	Blood vessel	Premature death	Regulates circulation
27. Amsaphalaka	½	2	Shoulder blade	Bone	Disability	Stimulates 4th chakra

Marma	Size in Finger Widths	No.	Location	Tissue	Effect of Injury	Effect of Acupressure
28. *Brihati*	½	2	Laterally from the vertebra below *amsaphalaka*	Blood vessel	Prema-ture death	Stimulates 3rd chakra
29. *Amsa*	½	2	4A above *amsaphalaka*	Liga-ment	Dis-ability	Stimulates 5th chakra
30. *Manya*	4	2	Side of the throat	Blood vessel	Dis-ability	Influences sense of timing
31. *Nila*	4	1	Throat	Blood vessel	Dis-ability	Influences sense of timing
32. *Sira Matruka*	4	8	Neck	Blood vessel	Fatal	Influences blood circu-lation in the head
33. *Krakarika*	½	2	Neck at the height of the shoulder blade	Joint	Dis-ability	Releases stiffness
34. *Vidhura*	½	2	Below the ears	Tendon	Dis-ability	Controls support of head
35. *Phana*	½	2	Both sides of nose	Blood vessel	Dis-ability	Reduces stress
36. *Apanga*	½	2	Corner of eyes	Blood vessel	Dis-ability	Reduces stress
37. *Avarta*	½	2	Above and at the end of the eye-brows	Bone	Dis-ability	Controls body pos-ture

Marma	Size in Finger Widths	No.	Location	Tissue	Effect of Injury	Effect of Acupressure
38. *Shankha*	2	2	Between ears and eyebrows	Bone	Fatal	Stimulates colon
39. *Utkshepa*	½	2	Above *shankha*	Ligament	Fatal	Stimulates colon
40. *Sthapani*	½	1	Between eyebrows	Blood vessel	Fatal	Controls hypothalamus (sleep and awake rhythm, body temperature)
41. *Shringathaka*	4	4	Palate	Blood vessel	Fatal	Stimulates nerves
42. *Simanta*	—	5	Suture of the skull	Joint	Premature death	Controls blood circulation in the head
43. *Adhipati*	½	1	Center of the back of the head	Joint	Fatal	Controls epilepsy

Asthi (Bones)

Susruta counted 300 bones, while Caraka counted 360. (Modern anatomy counts 203.) The difference lies in the fact that the former two authors counted teeth and cartilage. Fatty tissue (*meda*) forms bones from the elements earth, fire, and air. Classical texts distinguish between five different types of bones—*kapala*, or flat; *rucaka*, or shiny; *taruna*, or cartilagelike; *valaya*, or irregular; and *nalaka*, or tubelike (*Susruta-Samhita*, Sharira). Vagbhata mentioned that hair and nails are the waste products of bones. That leads to the conclusion that strong nails and hair are signs of a healthy bone structure, and that unhealthy hair and weak nails are signs of weakened bones.

Sandhi (Joints)

Tendons and ligaments, the body parts that hold the ends of bones together, are called *shandi*. The fluid responsible for the undisturbed movements of joints is called *sleshakakapha*. When *kapha* is disturbed, or when an excess of *vata* energy moves from the bones to the joints, different rheumatic illnesses result, such as *amavata*, *vatarakta*, and *sandhikavata*. In total, we count 210 joints. Of these, 68 are located in the extremities, 59 are in the trunk of the body, and 83 are found above the collarbone. They are divided into eight groups according to their shape.

Peshi (Muscles)

Muscles are different from muscle tissue, which was discussed in the second chapter. Although muscles are formed by tissue, they do not take part in any additional formation of body tissue. For that reason, they are called *upadhatu*. Ayurveda has counted 500 muscles. Together, they make up half of the body's weight. There are 400 muscles in the extremities, 66 in the trunk, and 34 above the collarbone. Women have 20 additional muscles—5 in each breast and 10 in the lower body. Muscle "fluid" (*lasika*, or secretions) helps muscles remain soft and subtle. At the time of death, the fluids harden, leading to rigor mortis.

Snayu (Tendons)

Tendons are formed from parallel, fibrous connective tissue. They are whitish at the ends and are attached to bones. Tendons are also called *vagu-vahani-nadi* to underscore their motor function. Susruta wrote, "Just as boards that make up a boat are glued together with different glues, allowing the boat to float in the water and to take on cargo, so is the human body held together by *snayus*." We differentiate between 900 tendons. There are 600 in the extremities, 230 in the trunk, and 70 in the region above the collarbone. Tendons are round, branched, or hollow.

Shira (Capillaries)

The numerous finely branched capillaries of the arteries, veins, and other vessels are called *shira*. There are 700 listed as important. They are further divided into those that carry blood, *vata*, *pitta*, and *kapha*. A cut for a phlebotomy is made according to this classification.

Pathology and Diagnoses
Nidana

The physiopathological characteristics of the three bio-energies, *vata* (motor), *pitta* (metabolism), and *kapha* (bio-mass) form the core of all life processes. We study bio-energies to identify substances with identical characteristics, measure the effects of individual bio-energies, and find healthy elements as well as those that cause illnesses. But what does it mean to be healthy, and what does it mean to be sick?

Health

To be healthy means that all physiological organs are functioning in perfect balance (*dhatu-samya*), that the individual is happy, and that all the senses (including the psyche and the spirit) constitute a harmonious whole (*prasanna-atma-indriya-manaha*).

Illness

We say someone is ill when he experiences pain (*dhatu-samyoga*). These sufferings can be physical or psychological in nature. The symptoms of an illness are signs that a disturbance is present. Symptoms present themselves in the three bio-energies, seven body tissues, and waste products.

Causes of Illness

Disturbances in bio-energies in *vata, pitta,* and *kapha* occur for several reasons.

Unsatisfactory Sensory Reactions to Stimulation (*Asatmyendriyartha Samyoga*)

The way the sensory organs react to input is of great importance for good health. The ability of bio-energies to balance themselves is diminished when sensory stimuli are too weak, too strong, or inappropriate.

An insufficient amount of stimuli (*hina-yoga*) is present when very small objects are viewed, while listening to almost inaudible sounds, when the tongue and palate receive insufficient flavors, when the nose is deprived of sufficient scents, or when the skin is deprived of touch.

Exaggerated stimuli (*ati-yoga*) are experienced with excessive noise, such as at rock concerts; with bright, gleaming lights; when spoken to with harsh words; when exposed to strong odors or unpleasant tastes; and with excessive pressure on the skin.

Examples of inappropriate stimuli (*mithya-yoga*) include viewing fear-inducing or very ugly objects, listening to ugly words or curse words, tasting contaminated or spoiled food, breathing unhealthy air, and experiencing unacceptable touches.

Exaggerated, inappropriate, and insufficient external stimuli have lasting deleterious effects, physically as well as psychologically.

Abnormal Behavior Leading to Inappropriate Verbal, Physical, and Mental Activities (*Prajnaparadha*)

The second factor causing illness is a person's behavior in relation to activities that support life and to the environment. These may be verbal, physical, or mental activities. Appropriate use of language, the body, and the spirit supports life and protects against illness. Inappropriate, excessive, or wrong behavior is considered detrimental and contributes to illness. The decision of what is right or wrong (or better yet, what supports or undermines a healthy life) varies according to each individual.

Abnormal verbal behavior is illustrated by lying, being argumentative, slandering, cursing (*ati-yoga*), a lack of communication, being taciturn, failing to express thoughts (*hina-yoga*), and by inappropriate, unnecessary, and excessive talk (*mithya-yoga*).

Examples of abnormal physical behavior include repressing natural bodily urges, gratifying those urges in a severe or untimely fashion, lethargy, overexertion and strained movements of the extremities, unnecessary fasting, excessive eating or eating at the wrong time, insufficient or excessive breathing, and unnecessarily prolonged breath holding.

Abnormal physical behaviors manifest themselves in fear, grief, anger, greed, vanity, jealousy, selfishness, prejudices, and indifference.

Effects of Climate Changes (*Parinama Kala*)

The third factor refers to changes in the climate, such as cold, heat, and rain, and to their effects on the bio-energies.

63

Hyperactive function of a bio-energy (*ati-yoga*) occurs whenever the weather is extremely hot, cold, or rainy.

Hypoactivity (*hina-yoga*) occurs when a winter is mild, a summer is not very warm, and when there is a lack of rain.

Malfunction (*mithya-yoga*) takes place when the weather is warm in the winter or cold in the summer (*Caraka-Samhita, Sutra-Sthanan,* and *Astanga-Samgraha*).

Body tissues (*dhatus*) are constantly dying as they are used up in the ongoing life-support processes. The potential deficit is made up by the intake and digestion of nutrition, which builds new tissues.

Health and illness are, therefore, directly dependent on nutrition and digestion. When digestion (*agni*) does not function properly, toxic substances (*amas*) are formed, rather than plasma (*rasas*). *Ama,* a blockage of body channels, causes the accumulation of bodily waste products (*mala*) and prevents them from being eliminated from the body as quickly as possible. This creates the first stage of illness.

Disturbed bio-energies also have a negative influence on body tissues. Bio-energies are aggressive; body tissues, however, are only reactive. If the disturbed bio-energies are stronger than the tissues' ability to resist, the illness will worsen quickly. But if the tissues are stronger, the disturbances are not as serious, and healing takes place rather quickly.

Four Kinds of Illness

According to the *Susruta-Samhita* (*Sutra Sthana*), there are four different classifications of illness.

Nija **(Endogenous Illnesses)**   These are internal illnesses, the result of disturbances of the bio-energies and body tissues. They are treated with medications.

Agantuka **(Exogenous Illnesses)**   These illnesses are the result of external influences, such as accidents, insect bites, injuries, and other violent events. They are treated surgically.

Manasika **(Psychological Illnesses)**   These illnesses are the result of emotions, such as anger, fear, anxiety, sorrow, and cruelty. Psychological therapy is necessary in these cases.

Svabhavika **(Natural Illnesses)**   These illnesses are the result of natural processes, such as aging, birth, and death. Treatment is subtle.

The Six Stages of Pathogenesis (*Kriya Kala*)

When making a diagnosis, it is important to investigate all the factors

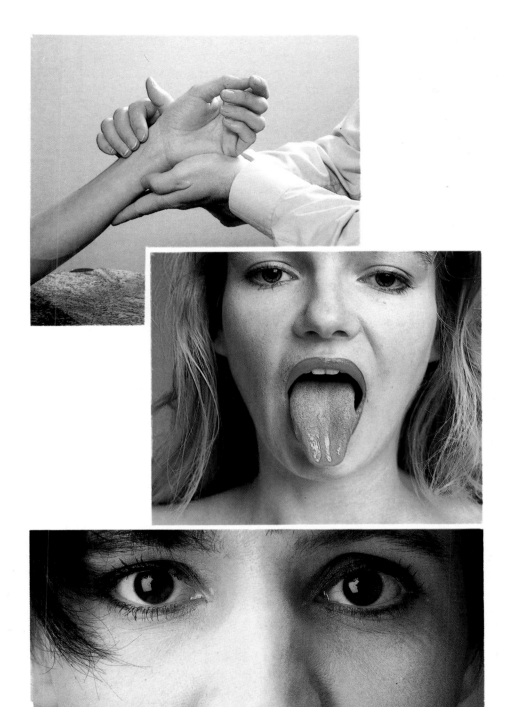

involved in the cause and development of the illness. All illnesses are caused by diminished bio-energies. In the beginning, they can be found in specific parts of the body or organs. In the later stages, additional signs and symptoms appear. Finally, they heal on their own, or they become more serious. Each stage takes a certain amount of time to develop (hence, the name *kala*, "time unit"). *Kriya* stands for the way bio-energies work. The course of an illness can be viewed as follows.

Sancaya (Accumulation)

A particular bio-energy may accumulate or become blocked at a specific site in the body or in an organ, meaning that the bio-energy has become hyperactive or begun to stagnate. In this state, the bio-energies cannot circulate freely through the body. The incubation period of an illness begins when a bio-energy becomes lodged in the body. The cause may be an untimely meal, a sudden change in the weather, or stress. Mild symptoms, such as a stuffed feeling (in the case of an accumulation of *vata*), slightly increased temperature, a yellowish coloration of the skin (in the case of an accumulation of *pitta*), a feeling of heaviness in the extremities, local swelling, or lethargy (in the case of an accumulation of *kapha*), will occur. If treatment takes place during this stage, additional complications can be avoided.

Prakopa (Provocation)

If enough bio-energies have accumulated, and if no intervention takes place, there is a tendency for the symptoms to worsen and for the illness to intensify.

Engaging in excessive athletic or sexual activities, carrying heavy loads, fasting, lack of sleep, and the repression of natural body functions lead to a provocation of accumulated *vata*. This bio-energy is strongest during cold and windy weather, early in the morning, and in the evening.

The bio-energy *pitta* is provoked by anger, jealousy, and fasting, by foods that are too spicy, too sour, and too salty, and around midday, midnight, and in the summer. In addition, frequent eating, particularly when the last meal has not been fully digested, aggravates the situation. *Pitta* automatically leads to a weakening of the blood. *Kapha* is increased by sleeping during the day, physical inactivity, and by heavy, sweet, oily, and fatty foods, particularly beef, pork, and shellfish. Symptoms are pain, flatulence, heartburn from sour substances, thirst, a burning sensation, an aversion to food, vomiting, and dizziness.

Prasara (Diffusion)

The effect of *vata* accounts for the outpouring of disturbed bio-energies, which leave their designated locations and spread out into areas occupied by other bio-energies. These bio-energies are then disturbed (alone, in pairs, or all three together). They begin (alone or together with blood tissues) to spread all through the body. There are 15 different possible combinations: (1–3) individual bio-energies; (4) *rakta;* (5) *vata* and *pitta;* (6) *vata* and *kapha;* (7) *pitta* and *kapha;* (8) *vata* and *rakta;* (9) *pitta* and *rakta;* (10) *kapha* and *rakta;* (11) *vata, pitta,* and *rakta;* (12) *vata, kapha,* and *rakta;* (13) *pitta, kapha,* and *rakta;* (14) *vata, pitta,* and *kapha;* and (15) *vata, pitta, kapha,* and *rakta.*

When *vata* is the main reason for the disturbance, swelling of the abdomen occurs. In the case of *pitta,* excessive heat might appear in particular areas or throughout the body. Disturbed *kapha* usually leads to digestive problems, loss of appetite, reduced mobility of the extremities, and vomiting.

Sthanasamraya (Localization)
As the disturbed bio-energies circulate through the body, they lodge in a place suitable for them. This stage signals the onset of an illness and justifies dividing illnesses into specific clinical groups. The symptoms point directly to the illness that follows them (*purva-rupa*).

If the location happens to be in the area of the abdomen, it is likely that internal abscesses will develop. In addition, there may also be reduced digestion, constipation, diarrhea, kidney stones, constriction of the urethra, incomplete urination, inflammation of the urethra, tumors in fatty tissue, pathological changes in the lymph glands, aneurysm (a pathological extension of an artery), scrofula (tuberculosis of the skin and lymph nodes), and elephantiasis in the lower extremities (an obstruction caused by congestion of lymph in the tissues below the skin). If disturbed bio-energies have spread throughout the body, illnesses will develop.

Vyakti (Manifestation)
Abnormal bio-energies now show unmistakable clinical symptoms and idiosyncrasies. This means that the patient exhibits an increased sensitivity to substances that are generally tolerated without causing any ill effects. The illness breaks out in full force and takes on specific forms (*rupa*); the tissues involved die off, and gangrene and necrosis set in.

Bheda (Termination)
In the last stage of pathogenesis, the process is interrupted and healing begins, or the illness becomes full blown. In the first instance, an abscess, ulcer, or wound breaks open, and the course of the illness is stopped; the body's own defense mechanism overcomes the illness. In the second instance, the condition becomes debilitating or leads to death.

In the first three states, where no specific symptoms are present, non-

67

specific treatment is initiated. Cleansing therapies (such as sweat therapy, fasting, and oil therapy) are used to stimulate the protective mechanism of the body. Such treatments are simple and should be undertaken as a matter of course, because in the later stages, it is often difficult to achieve healing.

Diagnostic Aspect of *Nidana*

In the classical texts of ayurveda, the chapter dealing with pathology is called *"Nidana-Sthana."* *Nidana* has three important meanings: (1) determining the illness, (2) investigating the situation, and (3) determining the cause of the illness.

The diagnostic aspect of *nidana* is divided into five groups.

Most Recent Reason for an Illness (*Nidana*)   The diagnosis leads to the reconstruction of the original cause responsible for the illness. Such a determination should be the basis for an effective therapy.

Warning Symptoms (*Purva-Rupa*)   The first signs are early manifestations, showing that a particular bio-energy is disturbed and might be the precursor of an illness. The symptoms are still very light and not very clear.

Clear Symptoms (*Rupa*)   These are unmistakable signs of the state of the illness. The symptoms are obvious and clearly show that a specific disease has developed.

Therapeutic Measures for Diagnostic Purposes (*Upasaya*)   Therapeutic measures are used when the cause for an illness cannot be clearly observed. The ingenious physician attempts trial therapy, which may include diet, medicinal, or physical applications. The physician observes the effects of this therapy to determine the appropriate bio-energy causing the illness.

Pathogenesis (*Samprapti*)   Pathogenesis means the origin and development of a pathological change in the body. After determining that such an event is in progress, an understanding of the precise nature and gravity of the bio-energies involved must follow. This has to include a determination of its location and the degree of spread.

If a physician begins to treat a patient without a proper diagnosis, any success (even if the physician is very competent in handling medication and therapy) remains purely accidental. Caraka set forth the prerequisite for a proper diagnosis: "A wise practitioner must use knowledge and intelligence to determine the internal state of a patient in order to arrive at a clear picture of an illness. This knowledge implies that the physician is an expert in his field, that he has a good intuitive sense, and that he is able to arrive at the proper conclusion." To reach such a diagnosis might take a lot of time, but it shortens the treatment time.

Three-Point Diagnosis
(*Trividhya Pariksha*)

In their writings, Vagbhata and Bhava-Misra describe the process of arriving at a diagnosis.

Darshana (**Observation**) The physician determines the gravity and extent of an illness and offers a prognosis. The first impression the physician has when introduced to the patient plays a vital role.

Sparshana (**Touch**) By touching the body of the patient, the physician can evaluate body temperature, the condition of tissues and skin, the patient's reflexes, and the degree of pain.

Preshna (**Questioning**) Through detailed questions, the different aspects of the patient's case history are established, including the physical and psychological state of the patient that a physician would be unable to find by himself.

Eight-Point Diagnosis
(*Ashta Sthana Pariksha*)

This system represents the classical form of clinical examinations in ayurvedic medicine. Since the thirteenth century, this has included the pulse diagnosis, which replaced the older, much more complicated and extensive *pancendriya-pariksha* (examination using the five senses).

Nadi Pariksha (**Pulse Diagnosis**)
Examination of the pulse (arterial flow) helps the physician understand the state of the three bio-energies. In general, *nadi* refers to tubelike structures or channels. Ayurvedic anatomy talks about 3.5 million of these channels in the human body, including the arteries. Pulse diagnosis is a science and an art at the same time. Arteries are like mirrors, reflecting health and illness, not unlike the way strings of a guitar produce sounds. The artery at the wrist (*A. radialis*) is best for this purpose. This type of diagnosis requires the physician to have tremendous powers of concentration and constant practice.

69

The examination includes determining the volume or quantity of the pulse, which depends on the bio-energy *kapha;* the tempo and frequency, which depend on *pitta;* and the rhythm and regularity, which depend on *vata.* The goal is to detect the predominate bio-energy (of one, two, or all three). Under certain influences, the beat (if *vata* is dominant) is like the crawling motion of a snake or leech; if *pitta* is dominant, the pulse is compared to the hopping motions of a sparrow or of a frog; if *kapha* is dominant, the motion is compared to that of a smoothly gliding swan or a peacock (*Sarangadhara-Samhita*). The motions can be specific and distinct, or two, or even all three, energies can be present together.

To determine the characteristics of the bio-energies, the physician uses the index, middle, and ring fingers. He uses the left wrist, if the patient is a female, and the right wrist, if the patient is a male. Both patient and physician should be seated comfortably, be free of stress and fear, and should have had an elimination of both stool and urine. The hand of the patient should be totally relaxed, held slightly at an angle, and not be too close or too far away from the physician. The physician lightly massages the hand of the patient with his left hand, holding the hand very gently. He then puts the aforementioned three fingers on the *A. radialis.* The pad of the index finger, which is positioned at the base of the thumb, identifies *vata.* The middle finger, which rests right next to the index finger, identifies *pitta.* The ring finger is positioned next to the middle finger and identifies *kapha.* A count of about 30 beats is sufficient; more can be taken, if necessary. The examination should be done three times with short pauses between each. The best time is in the early morning hours. The time of day, the season, hunger, any food eaten immediately before the examination, physical exertion, and different psychological states influence a pulse. These factors have to be taken into consideration.

The state of the subgroups of the bio-energies (*subdoshas*) and the body's tissues can also be investigated via a pulse diagnosis. Scientific research has shown that it is possible to determine the side effects of medication with a pulse diagnosis. Dr. K. Kodama has developed an instrument which identifies the *dosha* and the *subdosha,* opening up totally new possibilities in research and application. This diagnostic tool will be invaluable in the collection of medical and scientific data.

It is impossible to go further into the complex nature of the ayurvedic pulse diagnosis here. However, several extensive scientific projects are available to those who are interested.

Mutra Pariksha (Examination of Urine)

Early on, ayurveda acknowledged the importance of examining urine for diagnostic purposes. Although the method was very simple, it could be used anywhere and at any time without any technical device. The result of such an examination is sufficient for the experienced physician to make the right diagnosis. This type of examination and the resulting diagnosis still have legitimacy, because urine can be examined without a laboratory, and, if necessary, this can be done every day.

First, the patient is asked about the quantity, frequency, color, smell, and temperature of his urine. An adult produces about 1 quart (1 l) of urine within a 24-hour period. Since urine is a waste product of the body, elimination should take place at least six times every day. Any deviation from this norm indicates a disturbance. If *kapha* is hyperactive, the amount of urine produced increases. In the case of a *pitta* hyperactivity, the amount decreases. If *vata-kapha* is hyperactive, the amount of urine produced increases; in the case of *vata-pitta*, it decreases. Should all three bio-energies be involved, the amount of urine is very small, and the intervals between urination are very long. If the patient has a fever and a urine disturbance, the production of large amounts of urine is not a good sign.

Two ayurvedic standard texts, *Yoga-Ratnakara* and *Bhava-Prakasha*, describe the procedure of urine diagnosis. A sample of urine is collected early in the morning. It is important to make sure that the urine has not come in contact with the surrounding tissue. The urine is placed in a glass dish. Using a dropper, a drop of sesame oil is carefully placed in the center of the dish on top of the urine. If the oil disburses, the patient's illness is not serious and is easy to heal. If the oil remains at the same spot, it is an indication that the patient is dealing with an illness that will take a considerable amount of effort to heal. If the oil sinks to the bottom of the dish, it is a sign of a serious illness.

The way the oil moves (*gati*) indicates disturbed bio-energies. If the drop of oil moves on the surface like a float, or if it takes on the shape of a snake, *vata* is hypoactive. When the oil disburses into many smaller droplets and takes on the shape of an umbrella or a ring, *pitta* is disturbed. If the oil remains where it was dropped and takes on the shape of a pearl or a sieve, *kapha* is disturbed. If the drop sinks to the bottom of the dish, all bio-energies are weakened.

Vata disturbance is indicated when the quantity of the urine is small, but the patient urinates frequently. The urine is light yellow, thin, and somewhat foamy and cool to the touch.

Pitta disturbance is indicated when the amount of urine produced is not small or large, but urination takes place frequently. The urine is dark yellow, thin, and warm to the touch.

Kapha disturbance is present when huge amounts of urine are produced, but urination takes place less frequently. The urine is whitish, thick, fatty, and cool to the touch.

Whenever two or three bio-energies are involved, the symptoms described above are all present.

In days past, a high amount of sugar in the blood was detected by putting a dish with urine outside. If ants (present in all countries with a warm climate and known for their addiction to sugar) showed an interest, it was a sure sign that there was a high amount of sugar in the urine. Of course, today we have other methods for testing blood sugar.

Mala Pariksha (Examination of Stool)

If a person is healthy and eats properly, the food is completely digested. A healthy person's stool is solid, of sufficient quantity, light in weight (floats in water), yellowish, not too slimy, smells bad, and is eliminated without any strain twice a day. The color, quantity, shape, frequency, temperature, and possible side effects (all of which can be attained by questioning the patient) are important for a diagnosis.

Vata disturbance is present in cases of frequent constipation; where the stool is hard, dry, and consists of many small parts; is black or ashen; and when the patient has frequent urges to eliminate.

Pitta disturbance is present if the stool is yellowish or blackish yellow (less often green or black), watery, and mixed with blood. The urge to eliminate is increased, often accompanied by a burning sensation in the rectum.

Kapha disturbance is present if the stool takes on a whitish color, is mixed with slime and undigested food, has a less offensive odor, and there are frequent urges or eliminations.

Jihva Pariksha (Tongue Diagnosis)

The tongue diagnosis is the second most important examination. A normal tongue is reddish, supple, and clear, without a coating.

Vata hyperactivity produces a dry tongue, which is cool to the touch, rough, and with a reddish-brown coating. The predominate flavor preference is sweet and tangy.

Pitta disturbance is present when the tongue feels very soft and slimy, is dark red (in cases of acute infections), or is colored with a yellowish film. The patient has a bitter and sharp taste in his mouth.

Kapha disturbance is present when the tongue feels sticky and rough and has a white film. There is an extreme amount of saliva present, and the dominant taste in the mouth is sweet and salty.

Sabda Pariksha (Examination of Body Sounds)

Originally, only the sound of the patient's voice was listened to for diagnostic purposes. Later, a whole host of sounds emanating from the body were added. These include sneezing, hiccups, intestinal sounds, and gas.

The voice depends on the constitution of the person.

A person with dry air passages and a *vata* **constitution** or a *vata* **disturbance** has a dry, hoarse, shaky voice.

In the case of a *pitta* **disturbance,** a person's voice is rather loud and high-pitched.

In the case of **disturbed** *kapha,* the voice is not clear. The patient may interrupt his speech often due to mucous congestion. The voice has a low pitch.

Sparsha Pariksha (Examination by Touch)

In order to do an objective evaluation, the examining physician himself must be in good health. He begins by examining the different movements within the system, such as the pulse at the wrist and neck, the rhythm of the heart, and breathing. Next, body temperature, the condition of the skin (soft or rough), the joints, and the muscles are checked. In addition, he will determine if there is any numbness, paralysis, or atrophy (reduction in the size of organs or tissues). He will test to see if all reflexes are functioning normally.

In the case of a *vata* **disturbance,** the body of the patient feels rough and dry.

In the case of a *pitta* **disturbance,** the body feels hot.

With a **hyperactive** *kapha,* the body perspires, and the skin feels sticky.

Drik Pariksha (Eye Diagnosis)

Changes in the eyes point to malfunctioning bio-energies.

A **hyperactive** *vata* results in dry eyes. The eyes are set deep in the sockets. They are pink or covered with a grey film. The expression is one of anxiety.

In case *kapha* is **dominant,** the eyes are whitish, watery, shiny but without brilliance, and they seem immovable.

A **hyperactive** *pitta* produces reddish or yellowish eyes with a yellowish discharge at the corners. The person has an intense expression and is sensitive to light.

Akriti Pariksha (Observing the Total Appearance)

A person's total appearance correlates to his constitutional bio-type and depends on which of the three bio-energies is dominant.

Additional Methods of Examination

Other important criteria for an examination are described in the standard ayurvedic literature (physicians make use of them, too). Only after all relevant examinations—of digestive capacities, personal habits, resilience, and life expectancy—can appropriate therapy begin.

Digestive Capacities (*Agni Pariksha*)

Susruta has classified four groups of digestive capacities: (1) people with **well-balanced bio-energies** and good digestion, (2) people with irregular digestion caused by a **hyperactive *vata*,** (3) people with very intensive digestion caused by a **hyperactive *pitta*,** and (4) people with a very sluggish digestion caused by a **hyperactive *kapha*.**

Personal Habits (*Satmya*)

The human body is able to adjust to certain environmental conditions and personal habits, even those with negative effects. This holds true for eating and drinking habits, habits of behavior, and religious practices. For instance, sleeping during the day, because of the tremendous increase in *kapha* bio-energy, is very unhealthy for people with a *kapha* constitution or with a *kapha* disturbance. However, a person who has been taking regular naps after lunch for a long time will not experience any negative consequences. The same holds true when coffee and alcohol have been consumed on a regular basis. If the body and the psyche have become accustomed to them, no changes should be made. Therefore, before a physician has completed his diagnosis and initiates any treatment, he should clear these points with his patient, because lifelong habits influence the course of an illness and the reaction to treatment.

Patient's Resilience (*Bala*)

Bala, a person's physical resilience, must be examined to determine his ability to overcome illness, to predict the response to a specific treatment, and to predict the speed of recovery. This cannot be done by observing only external characteristics. For instance, we cannot say that a heavy person is strong, and a skinny person is weak. Therefore, eight essential parts (*sara*) must be evaluated. These include the seven body tissues and the psyche. If all parts are well developed, a patient will be able to withstand an illness. Should one or more be weakened, the immunity of the body is reduced. Accordingly, the goal of therapy is to built up the patient's body tissues and psyche. During the examination, it is also important to consider the age of the patient.

Life Expectancy (*Sadhya Asadhya*)

Finally, an individual's life expectancy is also taken into consideration when establishing a diagnosis. This is accomplished by using astrological calculations (*jyotir lakshana*); by interpreting the natural lines of the body, particularly the hands and feet (*samudrika lakshana*); by observing physical characteristics (*sharira lakshana*); and by identifying certain early symptoms in the patient (*arishta lakshana*). *Lakshana* is the term used to describe the aura of an individual. The ability to sense this aura or to learn the technique (and that of medical astrology) is discussed in other medical literature available to the practicing physician. This information can be very helpful. However, this should not be interpreted to mean that a physician, because of negative findings, should turn away or give up on a patient. A diagnosis must be based on medical and scientific knowledge. Information based on speculation should never be voiced to the patient. Only if the physician is an acknowledged expert in determining the aura of a patient can he use such information to strengthen the course of action he has decided to take.

Treatment Strategies
Cikitsa

Treatment is the practical use of medications or therapeutic measures to cure an illness. Its goal is to correct disrupted bio-energies and to preserve the balance between the three bio-energies—*vata, pitta,* and *kapha.* Ayurvedic treatment is prophylactic as well as therapeutic, because ayurveda is primarily a science of health prevention and only secondarily a science of medicine. The ideal is to prevent illnesses from developing in the first place. The chances for a cure are much better when an illness is treated in the early stages. To restore a patient to the original state of health becomes much more difficult and takes much longer when treatment is delayed.

Ayurvedic Principles of Treatment

Everything that influences bio-energies in any way—physical, emotional, or psychological—has therapeutic value. Indeed, one could say that nothing exists in the cosmos that could not in one way or another be used therapeutically. A story is told that the well-known teacher Atreya sent his students into the woods to collect plants without any medicinal value. When they returned at the end of the day, everyone except Agnivesha had picked some herbs. He explained that he had come back empty-handed because it was impossible to find anything that did not possess healing power in some way. The teacher was very happy with this answer and praised his pupil.

Ayurvedic treatment principles are divided into two groups.

General Treatment Measures

The goal here is to eliminate as quickly as possible factors that cause illness. For instance, for severe rheumatism and gout, meat consumption must be drastically reduced. But it is also possible that the symptoms of an illness are much more dangerous than the original illness itself. In both cases, a cleansing therapy will eliminate the toxic substances from the body and reestablish the natural balance of the bio-energies.

Specific Therapies

These are used according to the specific situation, which means that methods are used that promise to bring the best results. A distinction is made between treatment methods that are contrary to the cause of the illness, the illness itself, or both; and treatment methods that are similar to the cause, the illness, or both. Accordingly, this approach includes allopathic and homeopathic principles, as well as other healing methods.

Again, we see that ayurveda is a holistic medical system that is not separate and disconnected from medical science; rather it is an integral part of it.

Ayurvedic Principles of Treatment

General	Specific
Avoiding factors that cause illness	Contrary to the cause of the illness Contrary to the illness
Lessening symptoms	Contrary to the cause of the illness and the illness Similar to the cause of the illness
Elimination of toxins and *dosha*	Similar to the illness Similar to the cause of the illness and the illness

The Science of Medicine

Ayurvedic medicine distinguishes between irrational, rational, and subtle therapies. The rational therapies are further divided into dietary, medical, and life sciences. Medical measures are divided into two groups. In one group, no medication is used; in the other, medication is used. The nonmedication group includes physiotherapy and psychology. The group using medication distinguishes between internal and external use, in addition to surgery.

As taught in medical schools today, ayurveda includes only the rational, natural sciences (nutritional science, medicine, and life-style).

The other two aspects belong, more or less, in the area of philosophy and theology. Both are surrounded by a rather large grey area where, regrettably, many charlatans and dilettantes have taken up residence. This grey area has been partially responsible for the Western world's reluctance to accept ayurveda as a medical alternative.

Irrational Healing Methods

The so-called irrational healing methods include all those healing processes that elude human influence. For example, if a person is lucky, the illness goes away by itself. This could be called fate, or the belief that God is responsible for the healing. Endless reports of miracle cures have been around for as long as people have been able to talk. It is part of every culture, and it would be wrong to dismiss these healings out of hand. For this reason, ayurveda has integrated such "treatments."

Subtle Methods

As we all know, faith in oneself and faith in being healed can move mountains. If such an attitude indeed heals or minimizes an illness, ayurveda speaks of forms of treatment that have a mental or subtle basis. Healers without medical education treat people by the laying on of hands, telepathy, amulets, and similar methods. All these methods have one thing in common—they awaken and stimulate the power of self-healing in a person. The treatments include wearing precious stones chosen according to astrology; ingestion of precious stones and other tonics that, while they do not contain active substances, pass on the vibration of the respective elements; the use of color and *chakra* therapy; the use of mantras; doing "good works"; pilgrimages to specific locations that are said to possess healing powers; and the voluntary acceptance of sorrow in any form (renunciation or *tapasya*), so that involuntary suffering (negative *karmas*) in the form of illness might be influenced.

Modern medicine looks at these methods with skepticism or rejects them outright. Ayurveda accepts these methods because the cause of an

Ayurvedic Medical Science

Irrational	Rational	Subtle
Nutritional Science ——→	Medicine ←——	Life-style
Medicine without Medication		Medication and Surgery
Physiotherapy		Medication for internal use
		Medication for external use
Psychology		Surgery

illness can be found in such subtle factors. People who live very consciously and healthfully react very well to such subtle methods. For example, if you empty a bottle of ink into a dirty pond, the color of the water will be barely influenced. However, if you put a drop of ink into crystal-clear water, it will be noticed. Similarly, subtle methods are only effective in "clear water." A person full of toxins, like the pond, needs stronger measures. Use subtle treatments only as auxiliary measures.

Rational Methods

Ayurveda is unique in that it gives equal weight to diet, life science, and medicine. Each treatment, regardless of whether it is prophylactic or therapeutic, should include all three forms of therapy. The physician must convey the importance of adhering to all three methods. Our consumer-oriented society destroys almost all initiative. In the West, medicine has become a consumer product. Most people think of illness as a bothersome malfunction of the organism caused by circumstances outside their control or as the result of aging. According to ayurveda, this is wrong. Every person carries great responsibilities. Ignorance is no protection from consequences. It is our duty to adhere to the natural law and to follow instructions for caring for our psychosomatic "machine," the organism that carries us through life. The process of aging is influenced by how we take care of, use, or misuse our bodies. It is our duty to fight the unhealthy exploitation of our physical and mental strength and to protect ourselves from harmful environmental influences.

Most of therapy is devoted to diet and life-style, both of which provide protection in a prophylactic sense. Physician and patient should never lose sight of these aspects.

Medical treatment starts from the moment medication, surgery (when necessary), or non-medication procedures are initiated. In practice, these methods are often used simultaneously; however, they can be clearly divided into physiotherapy, psychological therapy, internal and external use of medication, and surgery. As far as the psychological aspect is concerned (the mental and spiritual side of the patient), conversations with a person that are holistically oriented and well-balanced, meditation, *pranayama* (breathing exercises), and *asanas* (yoga exercises) can bring excellent results.

Nutritional Science
Padthya-Apadthya

General Rules

Ayurveda does not have one diet. Rather, nutrition is extremely differentiated. Vitamins, calories, fat, carbohydrates, proteins, and trace elements can support or undermine health. What really counts is the energy of the food and its influence on the bio-energies. What is food for one person can be poison to someone else. The study of the elements, taste preferences, and bio-energies make it possible to determine the best diet

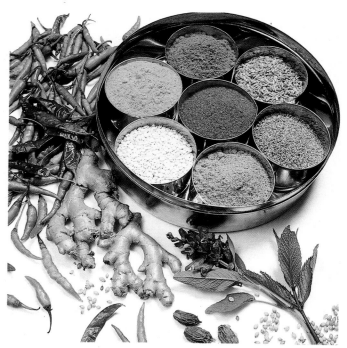

Spices play a central role in ayurvedic cooking. Added to foods, they can greatly influence the energy-giving quality of certain foods.

for an individual. The overriding principle is that the energies of the diet must be the opposite of those of the disturbed bio-energy or bio-type.

Improper nutrition is almost always the cause of a physical illness. Changing to a proper diet removes the most important cause of the illness. If the illness is not very serious, such a change can quickly lead to an improvement. Strictly speaking, nutrition should be approached on a long-term basis. Therefore, it should be considered part of prevention. It is important to remember that chronic illnesses do not become obvious until after many years of improper nutrition. Every organism possesses a balancing mechanism which corrects the effects of unhealthy habits as long as possible. However, one day these energies are used up and illnesses appear with a vengeance. The absence of unmistakable symptoms is no guarantee that a person has eaten properly or that one will be healthy in the future. Intensive care units in hospitals are full of people whose seemingly normal life-styles have been interrupted by a "sudden" breakdown. This is particularly true for diseases such as cancer, heart attacks, rheumatism, and diabetes.

Another often ignored factor is the influence food has on our psyche. Just as emotions influence the digestive process, so does the digestive process influence our psyche. This process is the basis of the effectiveness of the three omni-substances.

Foods with a Light Quality (*Sattva*)

Foods in this category open consciousness, bring the psyche to a state of harmony, and, eaten in proper amounts, do not have properties that cause illnesses. Light foods are fresh, juicy, oily, nutritious, and sweet. Wheat, rice, rye, milk, butter, honey, raw sugar, green vegetables, leafy vegetables, fruits, and nuts are included in this group. No more than eight hours should pass between preparing and eating these foods. At first, this might sound a bit strange, but the energy and consciousness expended while preparing food has a certain effect.

Foods with a Passionate Quality (*Rajas*)

Highly spiced, sour, salty, hot, and dry foods, such as hot spices, garlic, wine, beer, tea, coffee, cola, sodas, food fried in oil, salted bread, spicy food, and tangy vegetables all belong to the category of passionate foods. These foods stimulate sensual states, motivation, ambition, fantasy, jealousy, mania, and egotism. To survive in the world and to survive the constant demands made on us, we need a healthy portion of these passionate energies. A person who is fighting for survival can't afford to live as a monk in a cloister. His energy potential has to be kept at a certain level. However, in order not to burn up, the diet cannot consist of only passionate foods. It must also contain foods of a lighter quality.

Foods with a Sluggish Quality

Sluggish foods increase pessimism, ignorance, stinginess, greed, laziness, doubt, criminal tendencies, lack of good sense, and inferiority complexes. These foods require much energy for digestion. Included are canned and frozen foods; dry milk; root vegetables, except those that are sweet; grains that cause dryness; peanuts; leftovers and overcooked food; drinks with a high percentage of alcohol; and strong medicine. Meat and meat products are also part of this group, despite the fact that they have high nutritional value.

Other important elements are the time of day, seasonal changes, the frequency of meals, and the atmosphere during meals. Digestion is most active between 10 A.M. and 1 P.M., and the main meal should be eaten during this time. Seasonal foods should be preferred. They should correspond to the predominant, climate-conditioned bio-energies and consist of substances that are antagonistic to those energies. This subject is discussed in more detail in the Life-Style chapter. Regular food intake strengthens the organism. Eating between meals should be limited to times of hard physical work and then, only after the previous meal has been fully digested. Additionally, proper digestion is improved when eating occurs in a pleasant atmosphere.

A diet that is based solely on the bio-type is not always recommended. Other factors, such as age, gender, and those discussed in the last paragraph, should also be taken into consideration. Diets for elderly people should be anti-*vata;* for those in the middle years, anti-*pitta;* and for children, anti-*kapha.* Men should eat more of an anti-*pitta* diet, while women's diet should be more anti-*kapha,* unless other, very dominant bio-energies have been found to exist.

The cook asks how it is possible to do justice to every bio-type in his family. The question is justified. The answer is that bio-types are much influenced by heredity, or "the apple never falls far from the tree." Normally, bio-types are not that different within a family. In addition, by manipulating the temperature (from cold to very hot), using different spices, and serving the same food either raw or cooked, different effects can be achieved with the same foods. The amount of food served is also important. Ideally, a meal should include all six tastes. Together, they stimulate the senses and the production of gastric juices, lend a feeling of satisfaction, and prevent one-sided eating habits. Even an anti-*kapha* diet should not be without sweet, sour, and salty foods.

The following paragraphs describe in detail the diets for the different

82

bio-types. For instance, the goal of a *vata*-reducing diet is to tone down the bio-energy *vata*, meaning that it is suited for those with a dominant *vata* constitution or for those who suffer from a *vata* disturbance. Foods listed in the table Vata-Reducing Diet (p. 86) under Group A have a balancing effect that is stronger than those in Group B. Foods with negative effects on diminished bio-energies or bio-types are also divided into two groups. Foods in the X column can be eaten in small amounts now and then; however, they are not recommended. Foods in the XXX column should be avoided, since they are dangerous to the respective bio-energies.

Vata-Reducing Diet

This is the proper diet for people whose highest number of points was in the first column in the Bio-Type Test, that determines body type (see pp. 45 and ff.). These are *vata* people, or they have a *vata* disturbance. They are possibly undernourished; suffer from malnutrition; are constipated; suffer from insomnia, absent or irregular menstruation, loss of muscle mass, headaches, or impotence; are nervous or paralyzed; have dry skin, rheumatism, arthritis, flatulence, or cramps; are aging prematurely; and have many other symptoms or disturbances. For a *vata* person who has *vata* disturbances, this diet must be adhered to strictly. If only *vata* disturbances are present, but the constitution is different, this diet should be followed only until the disturbances are gone.

To soften the *vata* elements, ether and air, foods that are earthy, sweet, sour, salty, and have moistening qualities are preferred. Foods that are hot, bitter, and tangy are to be avoided. At least three regular, warm meals should be eaten. Ideally, such a person should never eat alone, and should not eat in front of the TV, or when nervous. It is good if another person does the cooking on a regular basis. People with very irregular habits, who jump from subject to subject, should adhere strictly to the diet. These people often suffer from food allergies, even from foods that are easily tolerated under normal circumstances. This is because they are hypersensitive. For these people, it is better to use ayurvedic medications rather than avoiding these foods. In general, fasting is not beneficial for such people, since it increases *vata* elements. In certain circumstances, a grape-juice fast (lasting for one or two days) and drinking warm water can be beneficial. Fasting for 12 to 24 hours twice a month is recommended.

Vata people need lots of water. However, water alone is not ideal, since it has no nutritional value. Milk and fruit juices are better, as are warm herbal teas that are calming and sweetened naturally. It is also beneficial to take a glass of red wine or 1½ ounces (30–50 ml) of ayurvedic herbal wine, such as *abhayarishta, aswagandharishta, balarishta, dantyarishta,* or *saraswatarishta,* before or with the meal. To assure that the body has enough vitamins and minerals, we recommend that ayurvedic strengthening medications, such as *cyavanaprasha, asvagandha lehya,* or *amalaki rasayana,* be taken regularly.

See the Vata-Reducing Diet table on p. 86.

Pitta-Reducing Diet

This is the diet for *pitta* people and for those who have *pitta* disturbances, such as most of the infectious diseases, inflammations, skin diseases, liver diseases, sour stomachs, diarrhea, high blood pressure, ulcers, etc.

Flavors that reduce *pitta* are bitter, sweet, and tangy. Spicy, salty, and sour foods should be avoided. *Pitta* people have a strong digestive system and can easily absorb food combinations with poor nutritional value. However, toxins (undigested food) wander into the bloodstream, leading to eczema, abscesses, acne, and other skin impurities.

A *pitta* diet should have a cooling effect. The *kapha* is well able to reduce the intense fire of a *pitta* person. Food fried in oil, highly seasoned food, and late meals should be avoided. Because of their susceptibility to liver diseases, *pitta* people should exercise caution when it comes to alcohol and fatty foods. Beer and red wine can be consumed, but only with a meal and in moderate amounts. Raw fruits and vegetables are very beneficial, but fasting increases *pitta* energy and should be avoided for that reason. A fasting day (supported by drinking apple, grape, and pomegranate juice) can be included in the regimen twice a month.

Pitta people need lots of liquids. Natural mineral water (without carbonation), sarsaparilla syrup, fruit juices, teas, and milk are beneficial. Strong alcoholic beverages and coffee are not recommended. Cool and sweetened bitter herbal teas are very good for liver detoxification. Thanks to their well-functioning digestion, *pitta* people can tolerate losing some vitamins and minerals. However, they do need calcium and iron supplements. Ayurvedic herbal wines, such as *ashokarishta, aragwadarishta, kumariasava, lohasava, parthadyarishta,* and tonics, such as *drakshadi leha, khadira leha,* and *satavarigulam,* are very beneficial.

By nature, *pitta* people are very emotional. For that reason, the atmosphere at meals must be calm. Family and business affairs should not be discussed while eating.

See the *Pitta*-Reducing Diet table on p. 89.

84

Kapha-Reducing Diet

If you are a *kapha* person or are suffering from *kapha* disturbances, such as obesity, a high level of cholesterol, dropsy, diseases of the respiratory system and sinuses, diabetes, gallstones or kidney stones, low blood pressure, and similar disturbances, this diet is for you. Walter and earth elements and their qualities (sweet, sour, and salty) are dominant. These flavors must be avoided. Food that is spicy, bitter, and tangy is the basis of this diet. Meals should be light, warm, and rather dry.

An accumulation of mucus in the body is always a sign that too many *kapha*-producing foods are being consumed. *Kapha* foods are primarily sweet. In practical terms, as little as possible should be eaten. Here is a person who will benefit from fasting. However, weight can be lost by eating from the group of foods that are listed in Groups A and B. The main meal should be eaten between 10 A.M. and 12:30 P.M. Breakfast may be eliminated, and the evening meal should be completed before sundown. If at all possible, *kapha* people should not eat between meals. In addition, these people should be careful not to ease their emotional problems by increasing their intake of food.

Under no circumstances should a *kapha* person take a nap after a meal. Also, the amount of sleep is directly related to weight. The more sleep, the greater the weight gain. Because of their physical structure, *kapha* types need very little fluid. It is a great mistake to think that because water has no calories, it does not contribute to being overweight. For the *kapha* person, it is important to take in as little fluid as possible. Cold drinks should not be consumed at all. Children and *kapha* people can get a head cold after just one glass of cold lemonade. Herbal teas with honey are ideal. Coffee and tea in normal amounts are not harmful. Milk should always be diluted to half-strength with water and should be consumed warm. The stimulating effect of white wine is beneficial for this type. However, even this should be taken in small amounts and only with meals. Beer and strong alcoholic drinks are not recommended.

Teas, such as *trikatu*, tonics such as *dasamula rasayana, cyavanaprasha,* and herbal wines, such as *vasarishta, parthadyarishta, dasamularishta,* and *pippaliasava,* are helpful.

See the *Kapha*-Reducing Diet table on p. 92.

Foods listed under Group A have a balancing effect that is stronger than those listed in Group B. Foods with negative effects on diminished bio-energies or bio-types are also divided into two groups. Foods listed under X may be eaten in small amounts once in a while, but they are not recommended. Foods listed under XXX should be avoided since they may be dangerous to the particular bio-energies or bio-type.

The *Vata*-Reducing Diet

Grains and Legumes

Grains are beneficial for reducing *vata*, but they should always be eaten warm or cooked. Dry cereals and breads made with yeast have negative influences and should be avoided. Most legumes cause flatulence, and they, too, should be avoided.

Group A   Wheat

Group B   Oats, Brown rice, Basmati rice, Mung beans, *Urid dal*, Tofu

X   Corn, Buckwheat, Millet, Rye, Barley, Granola, Chick-peas, Lentils

XXX   Dry grains, Cereals, Soybeans

Vegetables

Vata people can tolerate almost all vegetables. A diet consisting solely of vegetables, however, is not recommended. Many types of cabbage cause flatulence and should be avoided. Vegetables in the X group can be eaten if prepared with spices, oil, or ghee. Raw vegetables and salad should only be eaten when in season. These should be prepared with a sufficient amount of oil. Cooked onions may be eaten, but raw onions may not.

Group A   Sweet potatoes, Carrots, Parsley, Avocados, Radishes, Cooked onions, Seaweed, Red beets, Asparagus

Group B   Eggplant (Aubergine), Green beans, Artichokes, Fresh peas, Kohlrabi, Radishes, Watercress, Okra, Peppers, Cucumbers

X Potatoes, Cauliflower, Alfafa sprouts, Sunflower sprouts, Celery, Spinach, Cabbage, Brussels sprouts, Broccoli, Leafy salads, Endive, Mushrooms, Tomatoes

XXX Raw onions

Fruits

Most fruits are beneficial for *vata* types. A diet consisting exclusively of fruits, however, is not recommended, since, to a large degree, fruits consist of the ether element. Fruits increase body fluids; the exceptions are dried fruits, which cause flatulence.

Group A Lemons, Limes, Grapes, Strawberries, Cherries, Pineapple, Grapefruit, Plums, Pumpkin, Raspberries, Papayas, Mangos, Dates, Figs

Group B Bananas, Oranges, Peaches, Apricots, Garnet apples, Persimmons, Cooked apples

X Apples, Pears, Melons

XXX Dried fruits

Seeds and Nuts

Most seeds and nuts are good for an anti-*vata* diet. Because they are not easy to digest, they should be roasted with a little bit of salt and only eaten in small amounts.

Group A Almonds, Walnuts, Pine nuts

Group B Sunflower seeds, Coconut, Pumpkin seeds, Cashew nuts, Peanuts

X None

XXX None

Oils

With their warming and moisturizing qualities, oils are ideal for reducing *vata*. Since oils and fats are difficult to digest, their ideal application is external. For use in cooking, sesame oil is best.

Group A   Sesame

Group B   Olive, Almond, Avocado, Coconut, Mustard-seed, Peanut, Sunflower, Thistle

X   Corn, Soy

XXX   None

Spices

Spices stimulate the appetite and help to avoid flatulence. Practically all spices are acceptable on the *vata* diet. During the cold season, spices can be used more liberally; in general, however, it is wise to avoid very hot spices. A *vata* person needs a sufficient amount of salt.

Group A   Asafetida (*Hing*), Garlic, Cardamom, Nutmeg, Fennel seeds, Rock salt

Group B   Anise, Turmeric, Caraway seeds, Basil, Coriander, Cloves, Cinnamon, Ginger, Cloverleaf seeds, Peppermint, Mustard seeds, Saffron, Ajowan, Sea salt

X   Cayenne pepper, Chili

XXX   None

Animal Products

Fermented or enzyme-treated milk products are particularly good. Other types of milk are easier to digest when warmed or flavored. Meat products are best for *vata* people. They are ideal when taken in the form of a broth. However, when consumed over a long period of time or in excess, negative side effects, such as the accumulation of toxins and psychological disturbances, cannot be avoided. *Vata* people are particularly prone to these effects. In any case, vegetables are preferred.

Group A Clarified butter, Buttermilk, Milk, Yogurt, Kefir, Cream, Sour cream, Cottage cheese, Butter, Curd cheese

Group B Cheese, Fish, Shellfish, Eggs, Fowl, Turkey

X Ice cream, Beef, Lamb, Rabbit, Game

XXX Pork, Lard

Sweeteners

The sweet flavor of the elements earth and water have characteristics that are the complete opposite of those of *vata*. For this reason, a *vata* person needs sweets. However, refined, bleached sugar (particularly chocolates) is not recommended.

Group A Sucrose, Raw sugar

Group B Fructose, Candied sugar, Maple syrup, Molasses, Thickened pear juice, Honey

X None

XXX Refined sugar, Chocolate

The *Pitta*-Reducing Diet

Grains and Legumes

Almost all grains are suitable for this diet, since they serve to strengthen and balance the body without overheating it. Legumes have a more neutralizing effect than grains.

Group A Wheat, Mung beans

Group B Rice, Oats, Rye, Granola, Chick-peas, Beans, Soybeans, Tofu

X Corn, Buckwheat, Rye, Brown rice, Lentils, Millet

XXX None

Vegetables

Raw vegetables are very good for this diet. During the winter months, the vegetables should be steamed or gently sautéed in clarified butter.

Group A   Cauliflower, Alfalfa sprouts, Sunflower-seed sprouts, Celery

Group B   Broccoli, Cabbage, Brussels sprouts, Green beans, Leafy salads, Endive, Asparagus, Cucumbers, Okra, Pumpkins, Potatoes, Parsley, Fresh peas, Peppers, Eggplant (Aubergine), Tomatoes

X   Boiled onions, Carrots, Red beets, Spinach, Sweet potatoes, Radishes, Watercress, Avocado, Seaweed

XXX   Raw onions

Fruits

Almost all fruits can be eaten on this diet, since they contain a lot of water and have a cooling effect.

Group A   Apples, Garnet apples, Sweet grapes

Group B   Pears, Melons, Figs, Dates, Plums, Pineapple, Raspberries, Mangos, Sweet oranges, Raisins, Prunes

X   Lemons, Limes, Grapefuit, Sour oranges, Apricots, Peaches, Bananas, Cherries, Strawberries, Papayas

XXX   None

Seeds and Nuts

Salted and roasted nuts create heat, which is not desirable for this diet. Fresh nuts are a good source of protein and are to be preferred to animal protein.

Group A   None

Group B   Coconut, Sunflower seeds

X   Sesame seeds, Pine nuts, Pumpkin seeds, Almonds, Cashew nuts, Walnuts

XXX   Peanuts

Oils

In general, oils create heat and should be avoided.

Group A   None

Group B   Coconut, Sunflower, Soy

X   Olive, Corn, Sesame, Almond, Rapeseed, Margarine

XXX   Peanut

Animal Products

Milk products, if they are not sour or fermented, are well suited for this diet. All meat products produce *pitta* and are to be avoided. A *pitta* person has an ideal constitution for a diet of milk, milk products, and vegetables. These people can be very healthy without eating meat.

Group A   Milk, Cream, Buttermilk, Butter, Clarified butter

Group B   Cottage cheese, Salt-free cheese, Fowl, Turkey, Rabbit, Game

X   Eggs, Kefir, Salted cheeses, Yogurt, Sour cream, Curd cheese, Ice cream, Fish

XXX   Pork, Lamb, Beef, Shellfish

Spices

Use only mild spices. This diet should contain very little salt.

Group A   Coriander

Group B   Fennel, Caraway seeds, Cumin, Turmeric, Mint, Cinnamon, Saffron

X   Basil, Ginger, Nutmeg, Salt, Clover seeds, Asafetida (*Hing*), Cloves, Mustard seeds

XXX   Cayenne pepper, Black pepper, Garlic, Mustard seeds

Sweeteners

A *pitta* person needs sugar in order to harmonize emotions. Too little sugar creates irritability.

Group A   Sucrose

Group B   Raw sugar, Apple syrup, Fructose, Pear syrup, Candied sugar

X   Honey, Molasses

XXX   Refined sugar

The *Kapha*-Reducing Diet

Grains and Legumes

Grains that stimulate the kidneys and serve as expectorants are very good for this diet, but the majority of grains are not suitable. However, legumes are good. Tofu is the best source of protein on this diet.

Group A   None

Group B   Basmati rice, Buckwheat, Corn, Rye, Millet, Barley, Tofu, Lentils, Mung beans, White and red beets

X   Brown rice, Oats, Chick-peas, Soybeans

XXX   White rice, Wheat

Vegetables

In general, vegetables are good for this diet. A few, such as carrots and celery, stimulate the kidneys. However, eating raw vegetables is not recommended. They should be cooked with very little oil.

Group A   Celery, Broccoli, Cabbage, Carrots

Group B   Potatoes, Peppers, Cauliflower, Fresh peas, Red beets, Mushrooms, Spinach, Parsley, Asparagus, Radishes, Leafy salads, Watercress, Alfalfa sprouts, Sunflower sprouts

X   Onions, Tomatoes, Eggplant (Aubergine), Okra, Zucchini, Seaweed, Sweet potatoes, Cucumbers, Green beans

XXX   None

Fruits

Fruits contain a large amount of water, which is not recommended for this diet. However, they are also very light and do not have a negative influence on *kapha*, as is the case with grains and sweets. Therefore, fruits can be eaten in small quantities. Limes, lemons, and grapefruit are expectorants when consumed without sugar.

Group A   Apples, pears

Group B   Dried fruits, Dates

X   Plums, Garnet apples, Lemons, Limes, Grapefruit, Papayas, Pineapple, Oranges, Melons, Cherries, Figs, Pumpkins, Grapes, Mangos, Strawberries, Raspberries

XXX   Bananas

Seeds and Nuts

Seeds and nuts are not recommended for this diet, but they can be used as a source of protein that's preferable to animal protein.

Group A   None

Group B   Pumpkin seeds, Sunflower seeds

X   Sesame seeds, Coconut, Almonds, Cashews, Walnuts, Pine nuts, Pistachios

XXX   Peanuts

Oils

Basically, only the lightest oils should be used in this diet, and then, only in very small amounts.

Group A   None

Group B   Mustard-seed, Sunflower, Corn

X   Margarine, Sesame

XXX   Peanut, Olive

Animal Products

Except for buttermilk and goat's milk, milk products are not recommended for this diet. Often people have milk allergies. If this is the case, soy milk can be used instead. Meat, even when lean, is not suited for this diet. *Kapha* people need not be afraid that a lack of meat in their diet will be harmful. Rather than eating meat, it is better to drink a glass of wine or an ayurvedic herb wine. These will counter lethargy and stimulate the appetite and the senses.

Group A   None

Group B   Milk, Buttermilk, Low-fat cheeses, Soy milk, Chicken, Turkey, Rabbit, Game

X   Butter, Clarified butter, Kefir, Milk, Yogurt, Sour cream, Cottage cheese, Fish, Shellfish, Eggs

XXX   Pork, Beef, Lamb

Spices

All spices, particularly hot spices, are very good for this diet. Salt intake should be kept to a minimum and only slightly increased during the hot summer months.

Group A   Chili, Cayenne pepper, Garlic, Black pepper, Ginger, Cloves, Cardamon, Turmeric, Mustard seeds, Cinnamon

Group B   Nutmeg, Fennel, Mint, Coriander, Caraway seeds, Basil, Asafetida (*Hing*), Clover seeds

X   Salt

XXX   Refined salt

Sweeteners

Sweeteners are the most disturbing substance for *kapha*. Except for honey, which has a warming and drying effect, they should be avoided. Most *kapha* illnesses can be traced to an overconsumption of sugar.

Group A   None

Group B   Honey

X   Sucrose, Fructose

XXX   Molasses, Refined sugar, Raw sugar, Maple syrup

Life-Style
Swatha-Vritia

Health is greatly influenced by life-style. The goal of the ayurvedic life-style is to communicate generally valid information. We are not talking about moralistic finger pointing. The emphasis is on the influence behavior has on the bio-energies. The rules of behavior have been established to strengthen the immune system, which can make the difference between staying healthy and getting sick. Not all people who are exposed to the same germs actually get sick. The theory of ayurvedic bio-energy is very similar to the Western concepts of immunology and stress. No physician ignores the effects of stress, even if they can't be proven physically. The ayurvedic life-style teaches us practical rules of behavior that prevent bio-energies from being diminished. The body and psyche remain free of stress, which in turn strengthens the immune system and serves to protect us from illnesses.

Life-style is divided into four groups: (1) rules for behavior during the day, (2) rules for behavior during the night, (3) rules for behavior during the different seasons of the year, and (4) rules to prevent the suppression of natural urges.

Rules for the Day

Our daily routine begins when we awaken. The best time to get up is between 4 A.M. and 6 A.M. At this time of day, both the body and the mind are relaxed (assuming that you have retired early the previous evening). There is a saying that a *yogi* (a person who has committed his life to the spiritual world) sleeps six hours, a *bhogi* (a person who is happy to be alive) sleeps eight hours, and only a fool sleeps nine hours. If, for instance, you want to get up at 5 A.M., you should go to bed no later than 10 P.M. The habit of going to bed late and waking up late in the morning might create health problems, such as digestive disorders (dyspepsia), headaches, eye problems, and interruption of sleep (for example, to eliminate urine).

It is best to make a habit of going to the bathroom immediately after getting out of bed. If there is a problem with urination at that point, drink a glass of water or a cup of herb tea. Drinking coffee, particularly on an empty stomach, leads to pressure on the colon and eliminating stool.

The next step in the morning routine is mouth hygiene. Twigs from different trees are used in ayurveda to clean teeth. For us in the West, such a method is not really necessary—we prefer to use a toothbrush. What is important is the use of a sweet toothpaste for *vata*, a bitter toothpaste for *pitta*, and a tangy toothpaste for *kapha*—so as not to disturb the bio-energies. A *kapha* person usually has a lot of mucus that cannot be dissolved with sweet toothpaste. If all else fails, a bitter or tangy mouthwash should be used after brushing.

The next step is to free the tongue of its coating. A scraper, made from gold, silver, or a twig, is used for this purpose. In the West, this kind of mouth hygiene is almost unknown. However, if you have brushed your teeth and taken a look at what is coming off of the surface of the tongue, you will never ignore this part of mouth hygiene. Cleaning the tongue gives you a very fresh feeling, serves as the best prevention against bad breath, protects teeth from bacteria, and makes food taste much better. In addition, you do not have to use an overly strong toothpaste, which simply kills the mouth and throat flora, allowing those substances to reach the stomach and intestine. The last step is to gargle with cold water. During the cold season, warm water may be used.

Care of eyes comes next. They should be rinsed with cold water. Take a mouthful of water, open the eyes, and sprinkle them with cold water. Ayurveda also provides specific eyewashes. This procedure protects the eyes from hyperactive *pitta* and *kapha*.

Fingernails and toenails should be cut every fifth day. This should be done as part of the morning routine.

The human body must be exercised every day in order to enhance strength, stability, symmetrical growth, and the aura. Everyone has two kinds of enemies. The first are the external enemies (human, animal, or natural forces); the second are the internal enemies (diseases). A well-built body protects against both. Exercise cautiously, and only up to a certain limit, otherwise your health could be damaged. This limit is reached when you have to breathe through your mouth. Long, fast walks on flat ground, swimming, and yoga are ideal.

Exercising is followed by a massage to soothe the diminished *vata* bio-energy, reduce body fat, and to remove deep-seated deposits and dead skin. We differentiate between gentle and vigorous massages. Gentle massage is done with light strokes in up and down moves. *Vata* people use sesame oil, *pitta* people use coconut oil, and *kapha* people use no oil or a little baby powder. Vigorous massage is done with a massage mitten

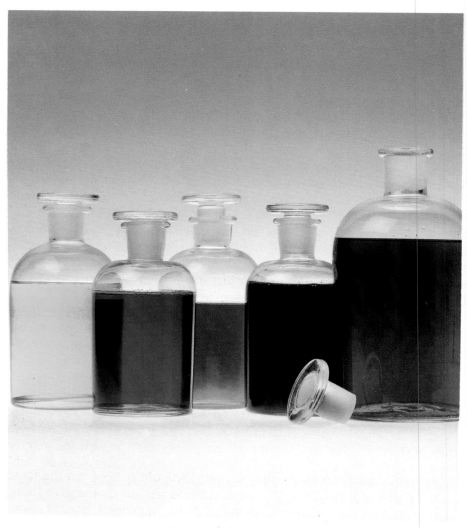

Photo:
Medicinal Oils (from left to right)—sesame, *balaswagandha thaila, prabhanja kudambu, pinda thaila,* and *gopadmajadi thaila.*

or a massage cloth. Both methods open and cleanse the pores of the skin, increase blood circulation under the skin, rejuvenate tissues, reduce fat deposits, and leave the skin glowing.

The oil bath can be given in combination with the massage or by itself. Of course, an oil bath does not involve sitting in a bathtub filled with oil, rather the whole body is rubbed with oil. You can choose from several different oils.

During the cold season, *pitta* people should use sesame oil instead of coconut oil. During the hot season, coconut oil is also recommended for *vata* and *kapha* people, instead of sesame oil. *Nilbringadi* can be used for all types in every season for both head and body.

Specific Oils for Oil Baths and Massages

Bio-Type	Head	Body
Vata	Sesame oil, *Nilbringadi*, *Kshirabala*	Sesame oil, Olive oil, Almond oil, *Dhanvantraram*, *Kshirabala*
Pitta	Coconut oil, *Nilbringadi*, *Triphaladi*	Coconut oil, *Candanadi*
Kapha	Sesame oil, *Nilbringadi*	Sesame oil, Mustard oil, *Thekaraj*

Choose a warm room with no drafts. It is best to put a large towel on the floor to catch any oil that drips. Warm the oil to body temperature in a water bath. Beginning with the hair, rub the whole body with the oil, including the feet. Do not let oil come in contact with your eyes; however, you should apply a few drops of oil in the ears and massage the inside of your nose with your finger. Feet, particularly between the toes, should be massaged vigorously. The oil should remain on the skin for at least 15 minutes, if time allows, up to one hour. In general, two oil baths a week are sufficient. From an astrological point of view, oil baths are best for women on Tuesdays and Fridays; for men, on Wednesdays and Saturdays. The positive effects are numerous. Most of all, an oil rejuvenates the skin and tissues, calms nerves, protects the eyes and ears, strengthens bones, and has a positive influence on the psyche. **Contraindications:** in cases of fever, directly after meals, after an enema, and during laxative therapy.

The oil bath is followed by a warm bath, including shampooing the hair with cool water (not ice-cold). Washing your hair with hot water leads to hair loss, premature greying, and is bad for the eyes. Instead of soap or shampoo, one may use simple, gentle ayurvedic alternatives, such as *mungdal,* chick-pea or soap-nut powder. All of these remove the oil, but do not damage the skin. However, you must be willing to put up with the additional work involved in the preparation and cleanup. Bathing twice a day is ideal. Baths not only remove dirt; they also revitalize the body, stimulate appetite, prevent itching and burning skin, and chase lethargy away. The best water is rain water, river water, seawater, or well water. The water temperature should be just below body temperature. During the winter months, you should not bathe in water that is too cold. In the summer, the water should not be too hot. **Contraindications:** fever, diarrhea, earaches, and immediately after meals.

After the bath, use a perfume with a natural scent. This increases the personal aura and strengthens confidence. Fresh, clean clothes, and jewelry made from precious stones increase the quality of life and provide protection from disease and negative influences. Such a start makes every day a special and unique day, because life does not begin at 5 P.M., or consist of only weekends and vacations. We live every moment, and that is reason enough to wake up every morning with the sense that this is going to be the best day of your life. Even a millionaire cannot afford to waste time.

If you do not take time for these small things, you diminish the quality of your life, your psychological and physical health, and your peace of mind. After all, we in the West know that it is the small things that make life worth living.

After bathing and after getting dressed, you ought to have a few minutes for quiet contemplation. The form of such contemplation—meditation, prayer, or just thinking of something beautiful—is a personal choice. Ayurveda makes no demands. It is only important that this time be spent in a quiet place without interruption. This process increases your concentration, strengthens the psyche, lowers high blood pressure, reduces hypersensitivity, and stimulates the resolve to take charge of your life.

What follows are a few tips on eating habits which were not discussed in the last chapter. In general, breakfast should be eaten before 9 A.M. and dinner before 9 P.M. There should be at least three hours between meals. Do not fast longer than six hours. Here is another piece of advice that seems to turn Western culture on its head—you should start out by eating something sweet (to reduce *pitta*), followed by something salty and sour (to stimulate digestion), and finish with something sharp, bitter, and tangy (to reduce *kapha*). The truth is that even in India, very few people adhere to these rules. However, in some instances, such as when the digestion is weak, this form of eating can be very beneficial. After a meal, it is infinitely better to take a walk than to stretch out on the couch.

It is important to drink enough water with every meal to stimulate digestion. If you want to maintain your weight, drink water during the meal; if you want to lose weight, drink water before the meal; and if you want to gain weight, drink water after the meal. Ideally, the contents of the stomach should consist of 50-percent food, 25-percent water, and 25-percent air.

Rules for the Night

Natural sexual activities keep the body vital, are healthy, and increase the body's aura. Form and frequency depend on age, physical condition, and the time of year. During the cold and dry season, intercourse is not restricted. During the spring and fall, it should be reduced to three times per week. During the summer months, it should be reduced to two to three times per month. After intercourse, a warm bath is recommended, followed by an application of fragrant cream, a few sweets, and a cup of sweetened tea, milk, or any of the *kapha*-stimulating drinks. **Contraindications:** incest, pregnancy, menstruation, with strangers, with the spouse of your boss, when ill, and with a much older partner.

The air in the bedroom should circulate freely. Sleeping with the windows closed is unhealthy. Because of the earth's magnetic field, the head should point either to the east or to the west. Sleeping on the right side of the body supports digestion. Normally, six to eight hours of sleep are sufficient. For health reasons, you should not sleep in the same room with animals. To prepare the body and the mind for a good night's sleep, try a few relaxing yoga exercises, a short period of meditation, or prayer. **Contraindications:** naps during the day, when obese, having a *kapha* constitution. (Of course, this does not mean that people with such conditions are not allowed to sleep; it only means that they should try to sleep as little as possible.)

Rules for Different Seasons

The twelve months of the year are divided into six seasons and into two halves, during which the sun moves towards the south or towards the north (*dakshinayana* and *uttarayana*), as described in the table below.

As the sun moves towards the south, its rays decrease. The cooling radiation of the moon and the water elements become predominant. All living organisms experience an increase in energy. The closer the sun moves towards the north, the more intensive the radiation becomes. This causes a loss of energy for all living beings. Changes from one season to the next are gradual and allow the body to adapt.

These changes can be the cause of illnesses. In ayurveda, the method of adaptation to seasonal changes is called *rutu-carya*, "the rules for the different seasons." It is recommended that you follow these three rules.

- **Balancing the Three Bio-Energies by Detoxification**
During the month of August, *vata* should be calmed by means of enemas; during November, *pitta* should be calmed with the help of laxatives; and *kapha* should be calmed in the spring by therapeutic vomiting.

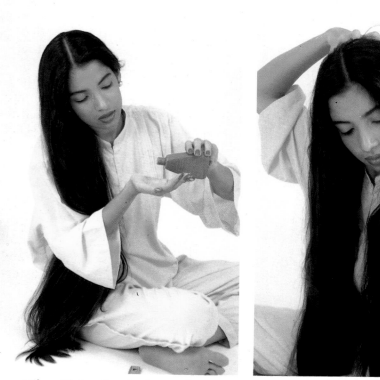
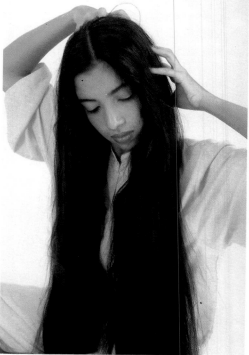

Oils with healing herbs, such as *Herpestis moiniera* or *Eclipta alba,* are cooling, promote hair growth, and protect the hair.

- **Diet Change** During the winter, early spring, and late fall, the diet should consist primarily of food that is sweet, sour, and highly seasoned. During the spring, the diet should consist mainly of bitter and tangy foods. In the early summer, the diet should consist mostly of sweet foods. During the fall, mainly sweet and highly flavored foods should be eaten.

- **Adaptation During the Changes of the Seasons** Periods of change occur during the first and last week of a season. These periods should be used to adapt to the new season ahead. Possible shifts in these changes should also be taken into consideration.

Six Seasons

Early spring	February and March	Sun moves towards the north
Spring	April and May	
Early summer	June and July	
Late summer	August and September	Sun moves towards the south
Fall	October and November	
Winter	December and January	

Early Spring—February and March

The nights during this season are still long, and, therefore, appetites are strong. Substances that increase *vata* should be avoided. A diet consisting of sweet, salty, and sour foods is recommended. In general, the diet should be much like the one eaten during the winter months.

Spring—April and May

Days and nights are equally long. This season is regarded as the first season of the new year. During the winter and early spring, foods containing oil and sweets have been consumed, causing an accumulation of *kapha* in the body. Due to the influence of the sun, these now melt and circulate through the body. This is the primary cause of digestive disturbances. For that reason, anti-*kapha* measures must be taken.

Increase physical and athletic activities.
Smoke herbal cigars, without nicotine.
Gargle.
Cleanse the eyes with eye wash.
Take hot baths.
Apply beauty masks to the face and body.

103

Maintain an anti-*kapha* diet.

Practice sexual intercourse.

Drink ayurvedic herbal wines, such as *draksharishta, durlabarishta, jirakarishta, kanakasava, mushtarishta, pippaliasava, saraswatarishta,* and *vasarishta.*

Use cleansing therapies (*panchakarma*), particularly those that include therapeutic vomiting.

Contraindications: sleeping during the day, fatty and cold foods.

Early Summer

The intensity of the sun draws moisture out of the earth and the bodies of all living beings. Direct exposure to the sun must be avoided, particularly around midday. *Kapha* bio-energies are reduced, while *pitta* and *vata* increase. All living beings have less energy. There are several measures to take during this period.

Food and drinks should be cool, sweet, and slightly fatty.

Alcoholic beverages should be diluted with water.

Pearls or pearl jewelry should be worn.

Sandalwood cream should be applied to the whole body.

The bedroom must be well ventilated and the body exposed to the rays of the moon.

Sarsaparilla syrup and ayurvedic jellies, such as *drakshadi leha, khadira leha, satavarigulam,* and *sukumura rasayana,* should be included in the diet.

Contraindications: physical activities, sexual intercourse, salty, sour, and highly seasoned foods.

Late Summer

All three bio-energies can be disturbed during this season; therefore, caution is advised.

Cooked food is preferred over raw.

Eat a well-balanced diet.

Sarsaparilla syrup and ayurvedic herbal wines, such as *kumariasava, lohasava,* and *punarnasava,* should be included in the diet.

Take oil baths and massages.

Wear light but warm clothes.

When indoors, stay in dry rooms.

Use cleansing therapy (*panchakarma*).

Contraindications: sleeping during the day, excessive physical and sexual activities, exposure to the sun.

Fall

Pitta energy that has been accumulated during the summer must be reduced.

Food and drink should be sweet and bitter and have a cooling effect.
Panchakarma, phlebotomy, and laxatives should be used.
Drinking water should be exposed to the sun during the day and to the
    moon during the night.
Indoor rooms should be decorated with fall flowers.
Fall flowers should be worn.
The body should be exposed to the moon during the early hours of the
    night.

Contraindications: eating foods that are difficult to digest.

Winter

As the nights get longer and the air gets cooler, *vata* increases. At this time of year, people develop a good appetite, enjoy good digestion, and have a lot of energy.

Foods should contain sweets, oils, and fats and be salty and sour.
Wine and other alcoholic beverages are allowed.
Oil massages and oil baths should be taken.
Warm clothes should be worn.
The bedroom should be slightly warm, and the bed should have warm
    blankets.
Sexual intercourse is suggested.
Athletic activities are encouraged.
Warm the body in the sun.

Contraindications: *vata*-stimulating foods, exposure to cold weather.

Regulation of Natural Bodily Urges

The repression of natural body urges plays a vital role in ayurvedic preventive medicine, since such repression can lead to very serious illnesses. Caraka wrote, "A wise person will not try to repress bodily urges that are felt from time to time." These urges develop through the downward movement of *apanavata*, located in the lower abdomen. If the urges are

Consequences of Repressing Natural Urges

Natural Urges	Illnesses Caused by Repression
Releasing Gas	Phantom tumors, flatulence, tiredness, colic, pressure on the heart
Stool Evacuation	Colds, headaches, burping, swelling
Urination	Tension in the groin, dysuria (painful elimination of urine), bladder and kidney stones
Sneezing	Migraine, torticollis (wry neck), facial paralysis
Thirst	Weakness, fainting, deafness, sore throat, heart pain, depression
Hunger	Dizziness, colic, weakness, skin discoloration, anorexia
Sleep	Physical pain, yawning, digestive problems, dizziness
Coughing	Increased coughing, breathlessness, lost appetite, hiccups
Panting	Breathlessness, phantom tumors, fainting, heart diseases
Yawning	Shivering, lost sensitivity, contractions, muscle spasms
Tears	Colds, chronic inflammation of the mucous membranes in the nose, headaches, heart problems
Vomiting	Breathlessness, itching, skin disorders, fever, swelling, coughs
Sexuality	Pain in the penis, vagina, and anus; urine retention; impotence

repressed, the corresponding bio-energies accumulate and cause disease by acting as pathogens. Thirteen impulses or natural urges are listed. When repressed, each one can cause health-related disturbances. (See table.)

In addition to somatic illnesses, psychological disturbances can develop that can eventually lead to psychosomatic illnesses.

Paying attention to physiological urges is a matter of hygiene, but the repression of mental impulses is recommended. Although the tendency to steal, insult, injure, or to have unnatural sex is human, exercising control is the duty of every human being.

External Cleansing
Bahih-Shodana

Ayurveda defines illness as the presence of a disturbance in the three bio-energies, *vata, pitta,* and *kapha.* The goal of therapy is to strengthen weakened bio-energies, to calm disturbed bio-energies, and to effectively maintain the status quo of balanced bio-energies. At the same time, the factors that cause illnesses have to be eliminated. Three different therapeutic concepts, internal cleansing, external cleansing, and surgery, make up the traditional therapies of ayurveda. This chapter discusses the external cleansing methods. These consist of external therapies, such as oil and sweat therapies. Depending on the type of illness, one external cleansing is sufficient. In general, this method is used before every *panchakarma* (internal cleansing) treatment. External cleansing opens up channels of circulation and moves toxic substances (*ama,* or undigested food) that have stagnated in the body, transporting them to a location from which the internal cleansing can eliminate.

The following therapies are only performed under the supervision of a physician. Several important factors, such as the levels of blood sugar, cholesterol, blood pressure, and liver function, must be considered. A physician observes the patient during the course of the therapy and intervenes if any contraindications arise. Most therapies must be performed early in the morning and on an empty stomach. Exceptions are specifically stated.

Oil Therapy (*Snehakarma*)

Sneha means "oily substance." Plant or animal fats are used. Sesame oil is the best plant oil because it calms *vata* without provoking *kapha.* It strengthens and protects the skin from diseases and fungal infections. Sesame oil stabilizes and warms and can be used as a vaginal cleanser. Of the animal fats, clarified butter is the best because of its particular compatibility and its ability to absorb medicinal substances. Clarified butter regulates *vata* and *pitta,* nourishes plasma and reproductive tissues, and contributes to a good voice and to the aura. Classical texts list over 100 prescriptions for medicinal oils. Some are still used today with great effectiveness.

The internal application of oily substances is discussed in the next chapter. These substances are preparations (*purva-karma*) for the *panchakarma* therapy, but they are considered as part of the internal cleansing procedure.

The therapies discussed in this chapter consist of 14 different external applications of oil. (See External Oil Cure table on p. 109.)

Oil therapy is recommended for: children, to support growth; later in life, to delay aging; treating dry skin; protecting against fungus; preventing insomnia; strengthening the immune system; anemia; dehydration; atrophy of organs and tissues; different eye diseases; insufficient sperm; excessive physical exertion; and balancing an unhealthy or excessive life-style.

Ointment Applications

For this therapy, the ointment is applied to the whole body. The physician determines the appropriate oil. Different oils can be used for the head and the body. Depending on the time of year, the oil can be cooler or warmer, but in any case, the temperature of the oil should always be above room temperature. Gentle circular motions are used around the joints. Care should be taken that the head, the ears, and the feet receive sufficient amounts of oil. Oils strengthen body tissues, protect against hyperactivity and hypoactivity of *vata* and *kapha*, soften the skin, and strengthen and increase the aura. This therapy can be performed every day, particularly for children and older people. The oil should remain on the body for 15 to 35 minutes. Afterwards, the person must take a warm bath or shower. In order not to remove all the oil, *shikka* or *mungdal* power should be used instead of soap.

Ointments are always applied before undertaking any additional therapeutic measures, such as pressure massage, foot massage, affusion, stroking, and treatment of the nose and ears. However, ointments can be used without other treatments. When no other therapeutic measures are planned, the oil can simply be left on to be absorbed by the skin.

Should the patient start to get cold during the treatment, he must take a warm bath. Ointments are applied in a sequence of six positions (see photos): (1) sitting up with legs extended, (2) on the back, (3) on the right side, (4) on the stomach, (5) on the left side, and (6) sitting up with legs extended.

The therapist begins with the first position. The oil is applied to the top of the head, towards the back (in the center), and covers all the scalp under the hair (photo 7). It doesn't matter if the hair gets oily. **Con-**

traindications: in cases of fever, constipation, extreme *kapha* disturbances, and after a cleansing therapy.

External Oil Cure

Ointment application	*Abhyanga*
Medicinal wrap	*Lepa*
Massage towards the heart	*Udvartana*
Pressure massage	*Mardana*
Massage with the feet	*Padanghata*
Affusion	*Parisheka*
Stroking	*Samvahana*
Gargling	*Gandusha*
Treatment of the head	*Murda thaila*
Treatment of the eyes	*Akshitarpana*
Treatment of the ears	*Nasatarpana*
Filling the ears	*Karnapurnam*
Head paste	*Masthiskya*
Bath	*Snehavagahna*

Medicinal Bandages

All infections and swellings should be covered. Depending on the desired
effect, different bandages can be used. Cool, absorbent, thin bandages
normalize *pitta* and the blood. Nonabsorbent bandages normalize *vata*
and *kapha* and reduce ulcers and pain. Bandages to which an astringent
healing substance has been added stop bleeding and dry out ulcers. *Pitta*
and *kapha* disturbances can be effectively treated with this method.

Massage Towards the Heart

In cases of *kapha* disturbances, obesity, diabetes, or dropsy, massages are
always performed with the stroking motion towards the heart. This is
particularly stimulating for the metabolism of the skin. In order not to
provoke a further increase in *kapha*, this massage is usually carried out
without the use of medicinal oils. Finely pulverized substances, however,
can be added. *Udvartana*, as opposed to *mardana*, is the only massage
that uses motions towards the heart exclusively.

Pressure Massage

Pressure massage (*mardana*) involves exerting pressure on the muscles
after or while the oil is applied. The amount of pressure varies according

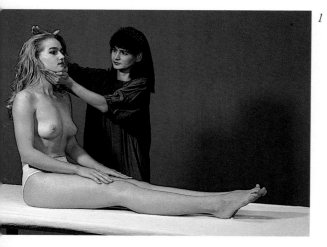

1

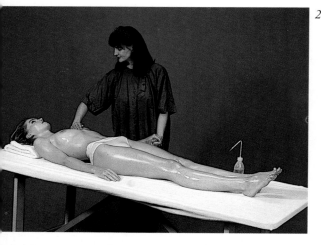

2

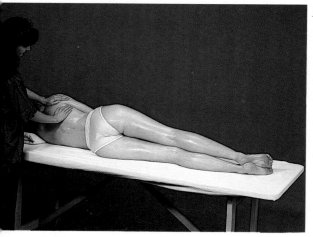

3

to the condition of the patient and the desired effect. On the one hand, pressure stimulates tissues and blood circulation beneath the skin; on the other, pressure has a tonic effect on vital points (*marma*). Furthermore, the therapist can address localized disturbances effectively. Pressure massage may be carried out towards or away from the heart. Since the main purpose of pressure massage is to regulate *vata*, it is carried out in the direction of the extremities. Depending on the patient's situation, two or four massage therapists can work on the patient simultaneously. When such simultaneous massage is performed, it is important that therapists apply the same amount of pressure (photo 8).

The massage is carried out with the patient in the same six positions as in the ointment therapy; however, it is not necessary to follow the same sequence. It is possible to combine both therapies.

The sides and the back of the head can be vigorously massaged using the fingertips, and the top of the head using the palm (photo 9). Posture is important. The patient should be sitting upright with a straight back.

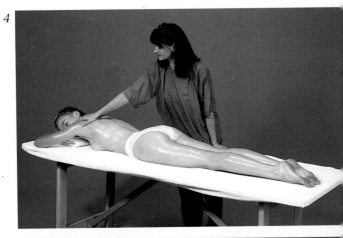

The next step is to apply oil to the back, breasts, stomach, legs, and arms so that the medicinal oils can penetrate the skin while other parts of the body are massaged. The therapist puts one hand on the throat, bending the head of the patient forward, while the other hand massages the neck region from the ear down (photo 10). While the patient bends his head back, the therapist holds the neck with one hand and massages the throat from the chin down (photo 10). Next, the head is turned to the left. One hand holds the chin, while the other massages from the ear on down (photo 11). This step is repeated with the head turned to the right.

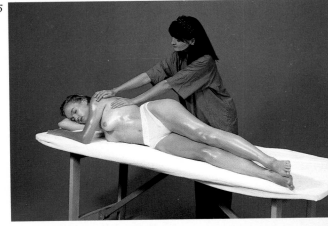

Massaging the shoulder and elbow joints is particularly effective with the patient in the sitting position. His arms should rest on the therapist's shoulders. Here, too, the therapist uses strong movements, massaging all the way down to the fingertips.

Now, the patient can lie down. First, the ears and the navel are filled with oil. Next, the vital points are

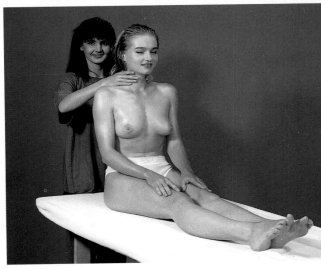

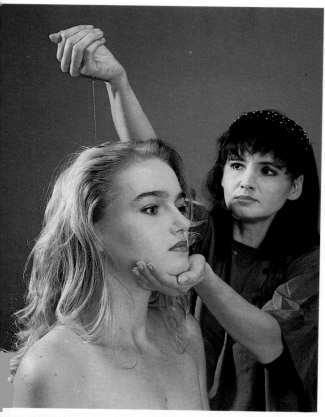

treated (see photos 12 and 13). Starting at the chin, the therapist moves with strong, slow motions to the back of the head, pulling towards the nap of the hair (photo 14). After the whole front of the body has been covered once more with oil, the vital points on the hands and feet are massaged (photos 15, 16, and 17). The therapist proceeds with long, strong movements from the sternum and shoulders to the tips of the fingers and from the hips down to the toes (photo 18). The stomach and abdomen are massaged with circular, sideways motions. The patient turns on his side, so that the shoulder blades, shoulders, hips, and backs of the legs can be massaged (photo 19).

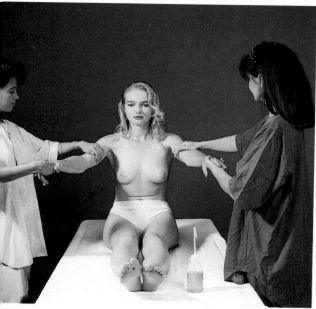

8

Now, the patient turns on his stomach. The head rests on the side. Halfway through this part of the massage, the head is moved to the opposite side.

If necessary, the head may rest on a towel. Beginning at the head, the therapist massages the back and the arms with even, strong motions, going down both sides of the spine (photo 20). Particular attention must be paid to all vital points in the lumbar region. Next, one leg at a time is slightly bent at the knees, and the soles of the feet and the ankles are massaged vigorously. The soles of the feet are massaged with quick movements using the flat of the hand (photos 21 and 22). The patient turns on his right side; the therapist massages the left shoulder blade, shoulder, and buttocks (photo 23).

To conclude, the patient sits up again (with legs extended) and breathes deeply. Starting at the neck and throat, the therapist moves one hand down from the throat to the navel region. With the other hand at the front, providing support, pressure is applied along the spine. Maximum pressure is applied when the patient inhales (photo 24). When the patient has finished exhaling, the therapist's hand should be in the navel region. Only slight pressure should be applied at that point (photo 25). Finally, the therapist moves his hands over the shoulders, arms, and elbows with gentle, short strokes. At the conclusion of the massage, we recommend sweat therapy or a warm bath.

9

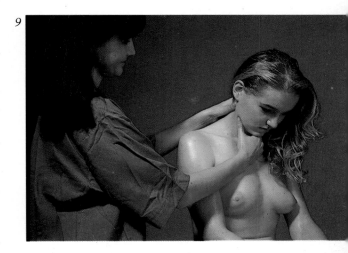

10

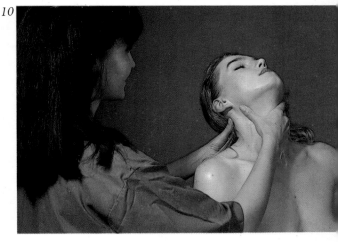

11

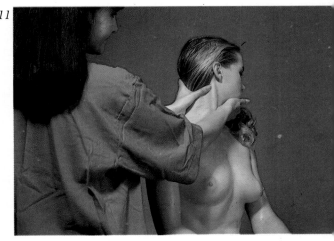

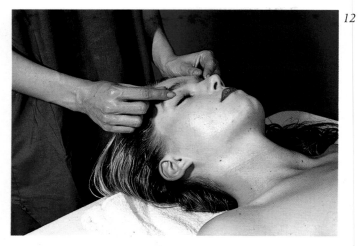

12

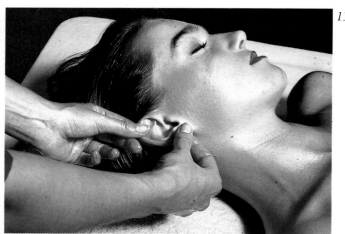

13

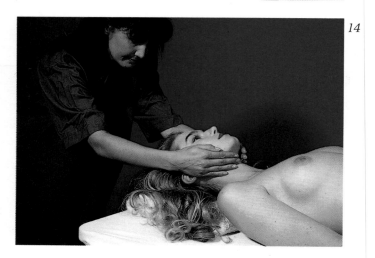

14

114

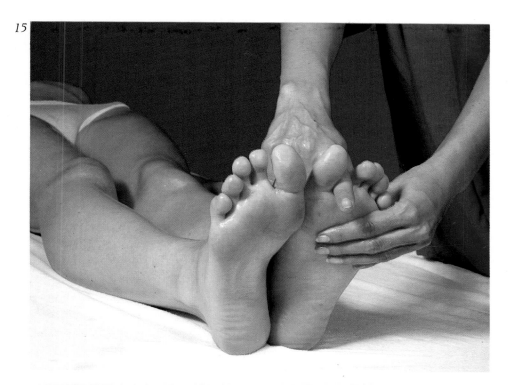

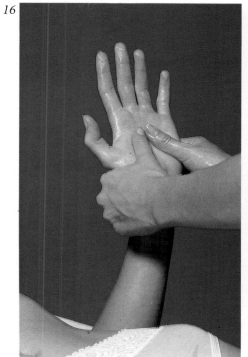

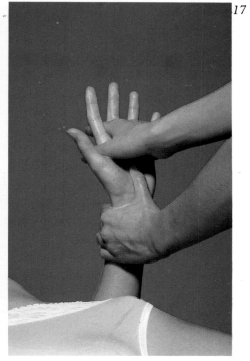

115

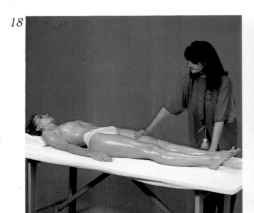

18

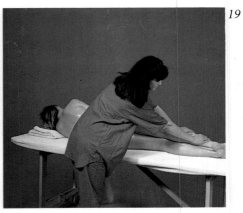

19

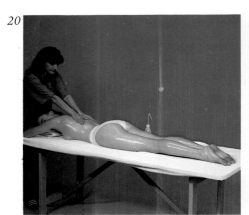

20

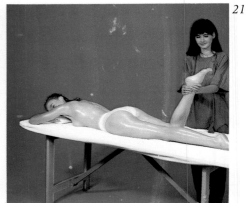

21

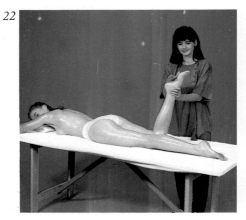

22

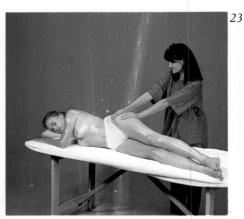

23

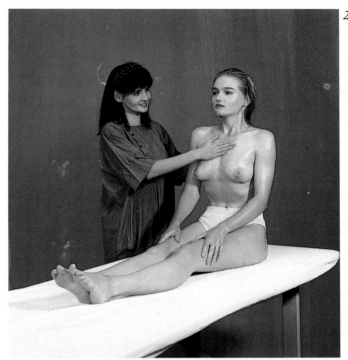

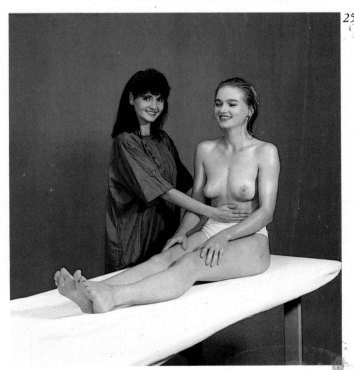

Massaging with the Feet

Today, this special massage method is only taught in Kerala in southern India, where a few schools teach the traditional martial arts. The method is used to make the body strong and subtle. Once a year, the students interrupt their training for a month and undergo daily massages using special medicinal oils.

Another type of *padanghata* was used by young, specially trained girls in "houses of pleasure." Men who were considered half-dead were brought back to life. This kind of massage was known as *malabarmalish*.

In ayurveda, this massage is used on patients in comas, in certain cases of mental illness, and for extreme *vata* disturbances. There is virtually no other massage that can claim such strong results. After the treatment, the action radius of the legs is much greater, and the legs are much stronger. In order for the therapist to maintain balance, he holds on to a cord that is strung above the patient (photo 26). The patient is first rubbed down with specially chosen oils. He then lies on his stomach with his arms stretched out in front.

A reed mat is the best surface for the patient to lie on. The massage

26

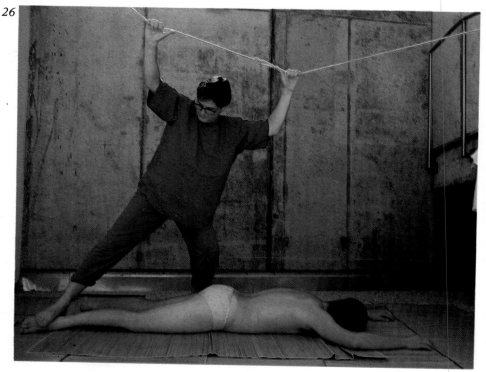

begins directly below the lumbar vertebrae and sacrum, moving up from there to the tips of the fingers and back down again to the tips of the toes. The therapist can move directly from the fingers of the right hand to the shoulders and the spine and down to the lumbar region. From there, he moves over to the left thigh and down to the toes. This procedure is repeated, starting from the left fingers, down the lumbar region, crossing over to the right side and down the right leg.

The effect of the massage can be heightened by having the patient assume specific yoga positions, such as the snake position (*bhujangasana*). He can then turn on his back with his arms still stretched out. The therapist uses the same procedure, starting at the front, where less pressure should be applied to the stomach, but increased pressure to the arms, shoulders, and thighs. At the conclusion of the massage, the patient must rest for at least two hours. Afterwards, he may take a warm bath and eat a light meal. The result of such a massage is a feeling of youthfulness. The patient is literally bursting with energy.

A regular ayurvedic foot massage is highly recommended for top athletes, people who are sexually very active, and for those who are very active in their jobs. Unfortunately, even in India, this type of massage is hard to find. In Europe, it is only available in the Ayurveda Clinic in Walzenhausen, Switzerland.

Affusion

Affusion is used in cases of *vata* diseases, for weakened conditions, and for bone fractures. It reduces pain from surgery, burns, wounds, and bruises. The liquid can consist of medicinal oils, milk, yogurt, buttermilk, clarified butter, or animal fats. Since the oil is usually heated and the patient breaks out in a sweat, affusions are part of sweat therapy and are discussed later in this chapter.

Stroking

Gentle, soft touching along the body's nerve channels stimulates circulation in these and other channels. Healing touches are sorely missing in our lives. The increasingly impersonal, anonymous atmosphere of our culture leads to isolation, particularly among the older population. This deprivation is the cause of many illnesses. Stroking should be part of every massage. It should be used at the end of the second position and up to the fifth. With the patient on his back, the therapist moves one or both hands in a constant motion over the right hand, shoulder, and breastbone down to the navel region, crossing over to the left side and moving

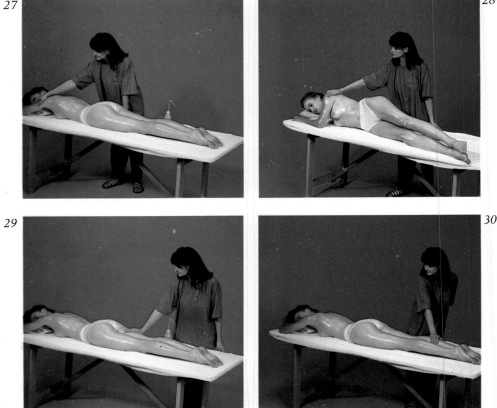

down the right leg to the toes. This is repeated on the opposite side. With the patient on his side, the therapist starts at the ear and moves down the body to the toes (photo 27). With the patient lying on his stomach, the procedure is the same; as soon as the therapist reaches the lumbar region, he crosses over to the other side (photos 28, 29, and 30).

Gargle

An ayurvedic gargle involves taking a large mouthful of an oily substance and holding this substance until the disturbed bio-energies have moved into the cheek area. Tears and a runny nose indicate that this has occurred. The procedure is repeated once. If no symptoms appear, it is necessary to experiment with different combinations of healing substances. The patient must sit in an upright position and must concentrate.

In general, gargling is indicated when the patient complains about throat, head, nose, or ear problems. Other indicators are tooth decay, toothaches, receding gums, neck pain, headaches, colds, and lack of appetite. The following healing substances are used for gargling therapy:

Sesame oil or clarified butter prepared with sweet, sour, and salty substances, such as herbs or minerals. These remove *vata* disturbances and are called *snigda gandusha*.
Clarified butter prepared with bitter, tangy, or sweet substances calms *pitta* disturbances and is called *samshamana gandusha*.
Clarified butter prepared with bitter, spicy, sour, and salty substances removes *kapha* disturbances and is called *samshodana gandusha*.
Clarified butter prepared with bitter substances heals ulcers and is called *ropana gandusha*.

The following reactions indicate the results of the treatment: Treatment was **successful** when the condition improves, when the patient has a sense of lightness and cleanliness in his mouth, and when he has an increased sense of perception. Symptoms indicating that the treatment was **not successful** are excessive saliva, weakness, and a disturbed sense of taste. Symptoms of **excessive application** are thirst, loss of appetite, dry mouth, tiredness, and inflammation of the tissues in the mouth.

Treating the Head

A head treatment requires the application of oily substances to the skull. These substances are allowed to penetrate the skin for a certain amount of time. Ayurveda distinguishes between four different treatments—*shiroabhyanga*, *shirasheka* or *shirodhara*, *picu*, and *shirovasti*.

Shiroabhyanga is the application of medicinal oils. Those that work best are *nilbringadi*, *kshirabala*, *anu*, *triphaladi thaila*, and *eladi coco* oil.

This treatment is indicated for hair loss, premature greying, thinning hair, fine wrinkles, and eye diseases.

Shiroabhyanga or *Shirodhara* reduces *vata*. Medicinal oil or other oils are poured on the head. A simple appliance, called *dhara patra*, is used. It can easily be made at home. You'll need two earthen flower pots of different size and about 1 foot (30 cm) of thick, cotton yarn. The larger pot should hold 2 quarts (2 L) of liquid; the smaller, 7 ounces (150–200 ml). The edges of the pots should be perforated, using pliers. The yarn is twisted into a wick that is pushed through the holes of the pots. The smaller pot is placed upside down in the larger pot. The yarn extends through the hole of the smaller pot and is tied in a knot. The wick extends about 6 inches (15 cm) beyond the hole of the large pot. This clinical instrument is very inexpensive, but very useful and effective.

The pot is suspended from the ceiling or from a bracket and filled with the medicinal oils chosen for the treatment. If *vata* is at issue, the oil is slightly warmed; for *pitta*, it should be cool. The distance between the wick and the forehead of the patient should be exactly the width of four fingers, approximately 3 inches (8 cm). The stream of oil should be as thick as the little finger of the patient. The patient lies on a table with grooves and a container for catching the oil (*thaila droni*). A bandage can be put over the patient's eyes to protect them. The oil should flow onto the forehead in an even, elliptical motion (photo 31).

31

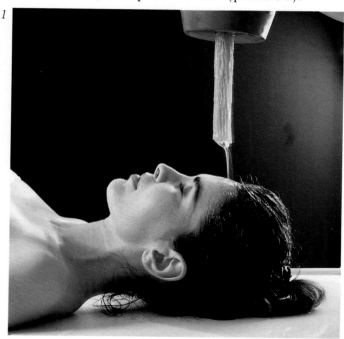

The first day, the treatment lasts for about 30 minutes. The time is increased by five minutes every day, until the maximum time has been reached. From then on, it is reduced by 5 minutes every day, until the time is 30 minutes again. Usually, head treatments are done without other treatments. However, they can be combined with affusion treatment, but the patient must remain on his back. The treatment is done in the morning between 7 A.M. and 10 A.M. on an empty stomach.

This treatment is indicated for chronic *vata* disturbances, such as migraine headaches, psychosis, signs of paralysis, apoplexy, mental illness, and insomnia. **Contraindication:** diabetes.

Picu treatment uses gauze soaked in oil, put on the forehead. The treatment is indicated for pathological hair loss, injuries such as lacerations of the skin of the head, inflammations, and certain eye diseases.

122

Shirovasti literally means "head enema." Since the skull does not have a natural opening, a leather cap is put on top of the patient's head. The cap is insulated with gauze. The medicinal oils are individually chosen by the physician. The temperature of the oil must be constant. This is accomplished by using a sponge to transfer it back and forth between the container and the vessel used for heating. The patient first should undergo a cleansing therapy suitable for his condition and, if possible, should shave off his hair before the treatment.

The treatment should be continued for seven days. It should be done around 4 P.M. In the case of a *vata* disturbance, treatment should last for 53 minutes; in the case of a *pitta* disturbance, 42 minutes; and for *kapha* disturbances, 32 minutes. For a healthy person, the treatment should last about 6 minutes. Whenever the patient's nose starts to run, the therapist knows that the treatment has been successful and can be stopped. After wiping all the oil from the cap with a sponge or a towel, the cap is carefully removed and the neck, back, and head are gently massaged. At the conclusion of each treatment, the patient takes a warm bath.

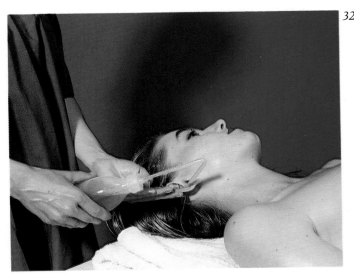

32

Treatment is indicated when a patient is insensitive to pain, has a paralysis of facial nerves, insomnia, or other illnesses of the head. **Contraindication:** the same as for oil treatments.

Treating the Ears

Ear treatment can be used daily as a protective measure for ear and neck pain and for headaches. Filling the ears with oil is a matter of course during every massage (see photo 32).

Treating the Eyes

This treatment can be initiated as a preventive measure, or it can be used to treat existing eye diseases. The patient should first undergo a cleansing treatment appropriate to his condition. The patient is on his back on a table. A 1½-inch (4-cm)-high dam (made from a flour dough) is built around the eyes to protect them. The patient keeps his eyes closed. Clarified butter is poured over both eyes until they are totally covered. After the liquid has been poured, the patient opens his eyes. The temperature of the liquid should be slightly higher than that of the patient. For a healthy person, and for those with *pitta* disturbances, the butter remains on the eyes for 200 seconds; for *vata* disturbances, 333 seconds; and in the case of *kapha* disturbances, 166 seconds. After the treatment is completed, the patient should not expose his eyes to strong light. In certain cases, milk or animal fats are used instead of clarified butter.

This treatment is indicated for glaucoma, cross-eye, trachoma, conjunctivitis, cornea inflammation, and night blindness.

33

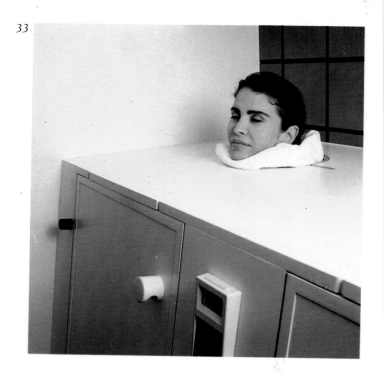

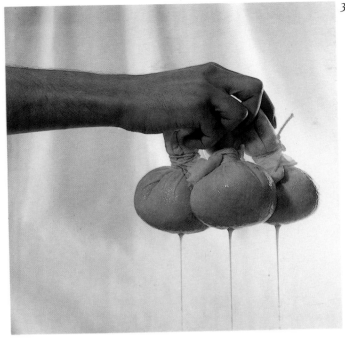

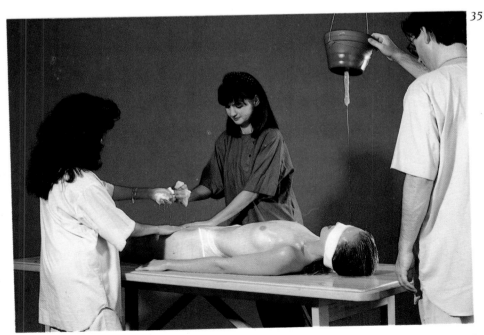

36

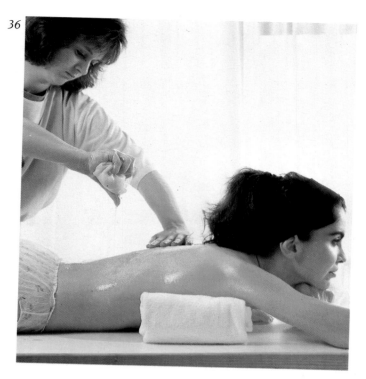

37

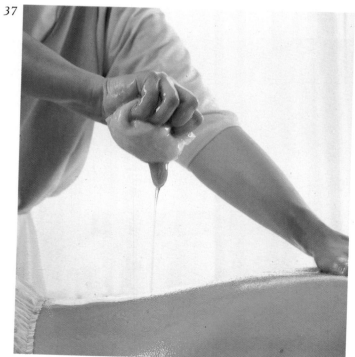

Head Creams

Strictly speaking, the application of medicinal pastes or creams to the head belongs to the section on medicinal bandages. However, here, special healing herbs and minerals are used for the treatment of brain injuries.

Bath

If you can afford it, you may sit in a bathtub filled with medicinal oils. Such a bath increases the strength and vitality of the whole body. However, this is not recommended for *kapha* people or those with *kapha* disturbances.

Sweat Treatment (*Swedakarma*)

Sweat (*sweda*) is considered a waste product of the body. If this waste product is not properly eliminated, several illnesses may occur. For that reason, sweat treatment, just as oil treatment, is both a pretreatment and a treatment in its own right. An oil treatment should always be followed up with a sweat treatment (photo 33) to eliminate sweat and other waste

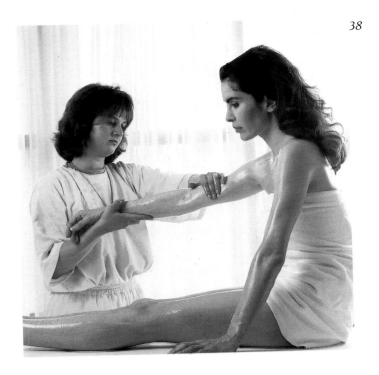

38

products, such as urine and stool. Sweat treatment is the best treatment for reducing *vata* and *kapha*. **Contraindications:** hepatitis, diabetes, vomiting, burns, poisoning, and diarrhea.

Indications that the treatment is excessive include muscle vibrations, trismus (cramps in the chewing musculature), a feeling of tightness around the heart, and dark coloration of the skin. If such symptoms occur, treatment must be discontinued immediately. The ability to recognize such symptoms cannot be learned from a book; it can only be gained from years of study and experience.

In general, ayurveda distinguishes between two different types of sweat treatment. The first type is initiated by "fire" (*agni*); the second, by physical activity, such as sunbathing, wearing warm clothes, and being hungry. Further distinctions include whether the whole or only parts of the body are exposed to the sweat therapy, and whether dry or moist heat is used. Caraka mentions 13 different methods (Caraka-Samhita, *Sutra Sthanam*). He describes the construction of the implements to be used, such as the steaming apparatus, sauna, heated stone plates, and how to create heat by fermentation, etc. Herbal steam baths are particularly useful for these therapies, locally or for the entire body. These use healing herbs that reduce *vata*, *pitta*, or *kapha*.

Professionals from Kerala distinguish between four methods—*thapam*, *upanaha*, *ushma*, and *drava*.

Thapasweda

For this treatment, gauze, towels, blankets, and such are heated and put on specific parts of the body. This is the method specifically used for the treatment of the mucous membranes of the nose. The patient always needs to be covered with a warm blanket during the treatment.

Upanahasweda

In this method, a warm paste (made of medicinal substances and liquids, such as coconut oil or milk) is applied to swollen or painful parts of the body. The paste is put on as soon as the patient can tolerate the temperature of the paste. The length of each individual treatment is determined by the physician. This method is used primarily for rheumatism.

Ushmasweda

For this method, dry or moist substances, such as legumes, rice, sand, salt, or cow dung, are heated, put into a gauze packet, and applied locally. In cases of chronic *vata* disturbances, the rice massage (*pindasweda* or *navarakizi*) is used. The procedure is to cook 18 ounces (500 g) of roots

128

of the *Sida cordifolia* plant (*bala*) in 10½ quarts (10 L) of water until the amount is reduced to about 2½ quarts (2½ L). This concoction is filtered. Half of it is mixed with cow's milk, and 10½ ounces (300 g) of navara rice is cooked in it. (Navara rice is grown specifically for medicinal purposes; it stimulates the regeneration of tissues). In the meantime, specially chosen oils are applied to the patient's body.

One half of the mixture is heated with an equal amount of milk. The boiled rice (divided and put into four or eight gauze bags) is heated in this mixture. Ideally, four (but at least two) therapists gently massage the patient with these bags (photo 34). The jellylike rice paste seeps through the gauze and is massaged into the patient's skin. The massage always begins at the neck and moves down to the feet.

Half of the rice bags remain in the hot liquid while the other half is used. The temperature of the bags is checked before they are put on the skin. As soon as they cool down, they are replaced with those that have been heated in the liquid. It is important that the bags be as warm as possible, but not so hot that they burn the patient.

The patient assumes six different positions on the table: on the back, the right side, the stomach, the left side, the back, and sitting upright.

Treatment should last 30 to 45 minutes. If the massage is done several days in a row, therapists should change places to avoid one-sided treatment. At the treatment's end, the bags are opened, and the paste is applied on the body. After a 5-minute rest, the patient takes a bath.

Dravasweda

Dravasweda is a method of pouring different liquids (milk, a concoction of healing herbs, or medicinal oils) over the entire body. The procedure for this well-known therapy follows.

Snehadhara (*pszichil* or *kayaseka*) involves pouring medicinal oils or other substances over the bodies of healthy people, too. The patient is first rubbed down with a medicinal oil (photo 35). The eyes are protected as shown. Approximately 4¼ quarts (4 L) of medicinal oil are slowly warmed to about 104° F. (40° C.). Four, but no fewer than two, therapists immerse pieces of gauze in the oil and squeeze it on the patient from a height of about 9½ inches (24 cm)—the breadth of 12 fingers. The stream of oil should be constant and as thick as a finger. The thumb points down to make sure that the oil flows in a single stream (photo 36). The application of oil always starts at the head and goes down to the toes (photo 37). Therapists use free hands for a gentle massage (photo 38).

The patient starts on the back and changes positions—to the right side, the stomach, the left side, again on the back, and sitting upright with legs extended. The treatment is divided equally between these positions. Sweat accumulating on the patient's face should be wiped away by the therapists. The treatment lasts 30 minutes the first day and is extended daily by 5 to 8 minutes. After the maximum time has been reached, it is reduced in the same way, until the original 30 minutes has been reached again.

At the conclusion of each treatment, the oil is removed with a towel. After a short rest, fresh oil is applied to the skin, and *rasnadi* powder is applied to the head. A dry towel, covering the ears, is wrapped around the head, and the patient is immersed in a bathtub to remove the oil. At the conclusion, the patient should drink a cup of hot ginger-coriander tea. If the patient is hungry, he may eat food appropriate for his condition. The patient should rest in a quiet place.

This treatment is indicated for all types of nervous disorders, hemiplegia (one-sided paralysis), paralysis, psychosomatic and rheumatic illnesses, after bone fractures, and as a rejuvenating treatment. **Contraindication:** diabetes.

Avaghaha Sweda treatment involves filling a tub with hot water and adding *vata*-reducing healing substances or warm oils. After medicinal oils have been rubbed into his skin, the patient is submerged in the water up to the breast. The temperature of the water must remain constant. A sign of a successful treatment is the appearance of sweat on the patient's face. This method is indicated in cases of hernia, hemorrhoids, chronic constipation, and stomach pain.

Kadivasti is a special treatment used when intervertebral discs have worn down and when the patient experiences hip pain. The day before the treatment, the patient takes a mild laxative, because he has to lie on his stomach for a prolonged period of time during treatment. Since this treatment is very similar to *shirovasti,* the same rules apply. After oil has been put on the skin, the patient lies on the table, facedown. A dam, made from a dough, is constructed over the lumbar region. Warm oil is poured into the dam. The temperature of the oil must remain constant.

Internal Cleansing
Antha-Shodana

Internal cleansing removes the cause of an illness and corrects the imbalance of the bio-energies. The cleansing therapy normalizes the physical constitution (*samshodana*) and calms bio-energies. It is used with medical therapies, special diets, and measures that support a healthy life-style (*samshamana*).

Panchakarma

Panchakarma therapy is the most popular *samshodana* method and occupies a prominent place in the classical literature of Caraka, Susruta, Vagbhata, and others. Until a few centuries ago, *panchakarma* was only practised in southern India and was almost forgotten. The enormous success of this form of therapy has caught the attention of the medical profession, and it has reclaimed its rightful place in medical schools in India. It has now been recognized internationally. *Panchakarma* is also viewed as an entirely independent treatment system, because it includes measures, such as phlebotomy (*rakta moksha*), that are really considered part of surgical procedures, as well as sweat and oil treatments, which are, of course, part of the external cleansing procedure.

Susruta divided *samshodanakarma* into three groups.

Purvakarma **(Pretreatment)** Every type of physiological cleansing requires strength and energy on the part of the patient. This procedure prepares the patient for the main treatment that is to follow. The goal of the treatment is to transport toxic substances that have become clogged somewhere in the body to places where the body can expel them during the cleansing process via the natural body openings. Pretreatment is divided into three sections—stimulating the digestion, oil treatment, and sweat treatment.

Pradhanakarma **(Primary Treatment)** This treatment consists of five different forms of cleansing that eliminate the accumulated toxins and waste products from the body—emesis (vomiting), purging (emptying the bowels with laxatives), treating the mucous membranes inside the nose, enemas, and phlebotomy. These five procedures gave this therapy its name, *panchakarma*, which means "five operations."

Pashatkarma (**Post-Treatment**) Depending on the goal of the treatment and the reaction of the patient, the main treatment is followed by different post-treatment procedures. These include diet adjustments, rejuvenating and health-promoting therapies, and calming therapy. In this chapter, we are going to discuss the five main methods of *panchakarma*. Pretreatment methods (external cleansing methods) were discussed in the last chapter. Ingesting substances, such as oils, and post-treatment therapies are discussed with the calming therapy, called *samshamana*.

Emesis (*Vamana*)

In ayurveda, the term *emesis*, or vomiting, is synonymous with the biochemical and biophysical processes that take place inside the body. Every author praises emesis as the most effective method of normalizing *Kapha* bio-energies, alone or in combination with other methods. In the *Astanga-Hridaya*, 22 different medications that initiate emesis are discussed. The experienced physician must choose among them, for instance, *Randia dumetorum, Glycyrrhia glabra, Lagenaria siceraria, Plumbago zeylanica, Elettaria cardamomum, Brassica campestris,* and *Acorus calamus.*

When *kapha* is the only bio-energy that is disturbed, plants that have tangy, spicy, and heat-creating qualities are chosen. In cases where there are *kapha* and *pitta* disturbances, those with sweet, warming, and mucous qualities are used.

After oil and sweat therapies, the patient should rest for one day. During the evening before the emesis treatment, he must eat *kapha*-producing foods. Therapy begins in the morning, but only when the patient feels hungry, because feeling hungry means that the previous meal has been digested. As soon as this takes place, the patient is rubbed down with oil. This is followed by a hot bath. An hour after the bath, the patient sits on a chair, and the stomach is filled to capacity with one of the following liquids:

Milk diluted with water, a small amount of potassium chloride, or sugar
Water diluted with milk that has been boiled with a small amount of rice
  flour
Sugar water or fresh sugarcane juice
A thin soup
Water mixed with a small amount clarified butter

132

The next step is to give the patient medication to induce vomiting, for instance 1 ounce (30 g) of *randia dumetorum*, ½ ounce (15 g) of *acorus calamus*, ½ ounce (15 g) of honey, and ½ ounce (15 g) of rock salt mixed together in 1 cup (240 ml) of hot water. Within the next 1½ to 2 hours, symptoms, such as perspiration, accumulation of saliva, and heartburn, should appear. At that point, the patient puts a finger in his throat and begins to vomit. Inducing vomiting before the symptoms appear is not recommended. Once the urge to vomit begins, it should not be repressed. In the interval, the patient should continue to drink diluted, boiled milk. When vomiting begins, the therapist should stand behind the patient, rubbing his back, sides, navel region, and forehead.

In case the patient throws up yellow liquid or small pieces of slime, the enemis should be stopped at once. If the content takes on rainbow colors or if blood appears, countermeasures have to be taken immediately. Vomiting will cease automatically if the patient stops drinking warm milk during the intervals. If the patient experiences pain in the neck, the stomach region, or in the sides, the therapist should rub *dhanvantaram kudambu* into those places. After a hot bath, the patient may eat soup. If the patient is not hungry, it is better to fast. A special anti-*kapha* diet should be eaten for eight days after the treatment. In the beginning, it should consist of only liquids.

If no vomiting occurs, additional medication must be given. The content of the vomiting is measured, but the first two are not counted. If the content reaches 2½ to 2¾ quarts (2.7 L), the treatment can be considered very successful; 1⅓ quarts (1.23 L) is considered moderately successful; but with only ¾ quart (.7 L) very little has been accomplished. The amount of medication given corresponds to the frequency of vomiting episodes.

Maximum (vomiting 8 times) is very successful.
Average (vomiting 6 times) is successful.
Minimal (vomiting 4 times) is less successful.

The patient should feel noticeably relieved. Vomiting first brings up the medication, then *kapha*, and at the end, *pitta*.

Purging (*Virecana*)

Purging, medically induced elimination of stool, is the ideal treatment for all *pitta*-related illnesses. It can also be used for *kapha-pitta* disturbances or for *kapha* disturbances that have become lodged in *pitta* locations. This treatment consists of cleansing the inner organs by eliminating stool. All classical texts list numerous medications that can be used for purging,

133

such as *triphala-churna* (*Terminalia chebula, Terminalia belerica* and *Emblica officinalis*), *Baliospermum mountanammell, Citrullus colocynthis, Citrullus vulgaris, Argemone mexicana, Mallotus philippinensis, Peterospermum aserifolium*, cow's milk, cow's urine, etc.

When choosing the medication, it is important to take the patient's digestive capacity into consideration. For people with a weak digestion, a mild laxative is sufficient. For those with a strong digestive system, more powerful medication should be chosen. Giving smaller doses in short intervals is preferred to large doses given all at once. The recommended medication is *avipathi churnam*. It is best given during the so-called *pittakala*, a time when *pitta* is dominant. The patient is not allowed to eat until the cleansing is completed, which, under normal circumstances, takes about 12 hours. When the medication is taken by midnight, the patient can eat again at noon the next day.

Oil and sweat therapies are a must before purging. For hepatitis, diabetes, trauma, edema, chronic abscesses, and anemia, pretreatment should be kept to a minimum. If the laxative has not been effective, the patient may eat a light meal. The process is repeated the next day with a different or modified dose until success is achieved. Drinking warm water during the treatment stimulates evacuation of stool.

The patient is well cleansed when he has 30 eliminations, moderately cleansed with 20 eliminations, and poorly cleansed when he has 10 eliminations.

Therapy must be discontinued when slime is detected in the stool, and the patient must go on an eight-day anti-*kapha* diet. If a patient needs both emesis and purging therapy, emesis therapy is performed first. In order to regain strength for the purging therapy, the patient should follow an anti-*kapha* diet that contains highly nutritious food. Purging therapy can be started five days after the emesis therapy. Three days before purging is to commence, the patient undergoes oil therapy. **Contraindications:** injuries to the rectum, diarrhea, and after the patient has had an enema.

Therapy of the Nasal Mucous Membrane (*Nasya*)

The application of medicinal oils or powders via the nose is called *nasya*. This is an ideal method for administering prescription medication for illnesses of the head. One method, which can be used daily and at any time of the year, consists of dipping a finger into oil and massaging the inside of the nose. This method provides effective protection against colds and prevents the mucous membranes from drying out. When the mucous membranes of the nose are to be treated, oil therapy should not be used

134

beforehand. After a patient has finished his morning routine, he should eat breakfast and thoroughly cleanse his teeth and mouth. The nose and throat can be cleaned by smoking an herbal cigar or a pipe filled with specific healing herbs. The patient may inhale through the nose or the mouth, but he should exhale only through the mouth. The next step is to massage the head and throat with *kshirabala* oil. This is followed by an application of *thapasweda* (with a warm gauze cloth) to the forehead, cheeks, throat, and chin. The patient lies down on his back with his head slightly bent back. The oil, which has been warmed in a water bath, is placed into both nostrils. Oil that runs into the mouth can be spat out. During this procedure, gently massage the hands, feet, and shoulders followed by repetition of *thapasweda* to the appropriate body parts.

The amount of oil used depends on the degree of the illness and the medication used. It varies between 2 and 64 drops.

For certain *kapha* disturbances, medicinal powders are used instead of oil. The patient can inhale the powder into the nose, or the therapist can blow the powder into the patient's nose. The preparation of the patient is the same as the one described above.

At the end of treatment, the patient should drink hot water and eat an anti-*kapha* diet. The patient is not allowed to nap during the day.

Enema (*Vasti*)

The name *vasti* comes from the bladder of the buffalo, originally used for this treatment. The bladder was filled with different liquids. Depending on what part of the intestine was to be treated, attachments of different lengths, widths, and shapes were used. The great advantage was that the therapist could precisely gauge the pressure. He could also detect the counterpressure. Today, this procedure has been replaced by syringes that can be attached to the hose of the enema bag.

This type of enema is the most effective method for treating *vata* disturbances. It is the cleansing therapy most often used. It is different in several respects from the modern enemas used today. In ayurvedic medicine, enema therapy is cleansing when used with *samshodana* (a cleansing medication). This medication lessens the symptoms and strengthens the body, if substances are used that support certain tissues.

Ayurveda differentiates among rectal enemas, urethral enemas, vaginal enemas, or other openings, such as abscesses. In addition, we distinguish between *niruha vasti* and *kashaya vasti* (enemas using liquids prepared with different healing substances) and *sneha vasti* (enemas using oily substances). Regardless of what is used, the patient is prepared by undergoing an oil therapy or a sweat therapy.

135

Enemas Using Oily Substances

In general, oily substances should remain in the intestines for nine hours before being expelled. In special cases, they may remain in the intestines for 24 hours. If no evacuation takes place naturally after that time, the patient is given a laxative. The amount of the oil-containing substance used is ⅓ to 1 cup (80 to 240 ml). This treatment can be used daily for some time, since it has rejuvenating properties and strengthens the body and the metabolism. **Contraindications:** in cases of skin disorders, diabetes, obesity, worm infection, loss of appetite, gout, and hepatitis.

Enemas Using Liquids Made with Healing Herbs

Enema therapy using herbal solutions is cleansing. In general, it should be used after an oil enema to prevent the intestines from drying out. Usually, herbal solutions with sour characteristics are used. Other solutions include mixtures of milk, honey, herbs, and oils. In cases of chronic constipation, a combination of 4 ounces (120 ml) of milk, 2 ounces (60 ml) of castor oil, ⅔ ounce (20 ml) of honey, and ¼ ounce (6 g) of *saindava* (a natural mineral salt) is recommended. This enema should not remain in the intestines for longer than 45 minutes. The enema first produces feces, followed by bile, and lastly mucous matter. The patient should feel light, not weak, after the treatment.

Treatment is indicated for kidney stones, gout, constipation, nervousness, loss of appetite, headaches, and heart diseases. **Contraindications:** cough, hemorrhoids, injuries to the anus, diabetes, obesity, and after purging or nose therapy.

Phlebotomy (*Rakta Moksha*)

Rakta moksha literally means "releasing blood." It is done by vein sectioning, blood leeches, a bell-shaped suctioning cup, or a horn. If the disturbances of the blood are due to *vata,* a horn is recommended. This method has a warming and calming effect. The skin is cut lightly, and the horn from a buffalo or a cow is placed over the cut. The physician then draws the blood by sucking at the thin, opposite end.

If the blood disturbance is caused by *pitta,* leeches, which have cooling and sweet properties, are used. If the disturbance is caused by *kapha,* the bell-shaped suction cup is used. This cup is made from a pumpkin, which has an irritating, tangy, and heating effect.

Vein sectioning is used when larger amounts of blood have to be extracted from the system. The cut is made with a surgical instrument. The direction of the cut should always be made in an upward direction so as not to restrict the flow of the blood. Each cut should be used only once, and care must be taken to avoid the vicinity of vital points.

136

The use of leeches is recommended for gout, hemorrhoids, certain throat and eye diseases, abscesses, tetanus, migraine headaches, hysteria, liver and spleen enlargements, and erysipelas. Approximately six different types of leeches are available. Before they are applied to the skin, the leeches are cleaned by putting them first in water and *kurkuma*, then in diluted milk, and lastly in water. Only then are they to be put on the respective part of the body. It is said that leeches will first draw out toxic blood, only when "clean" blood is drawn out will the patient feel itching or pain. At the conclusion of treatment, the leeches can be easily removed from the skin by sprinkling a little salt around the opening of the leeches' mouths. Today, in the age of AIDS, this treatment is not without risk, and, therefore, it is not recommended. Instead, sterile surgical instruments used in a clinical setting are preferred. **Contraindication:** asthma, pregnancy, cough, when vomiting blood, dropsy, anemia, for children under the age of 16, and for people over 70.

Calming Therapies (*Samshamana*)

Samshamana, or calming therapies, combine medication and diet with recommendations concerning life-style. Ayurveda uses medications that promote digestion and diets that promote digestion, medications that increase appetite and diets that promote appetite, fasting, decreasing fluid intake, physical activity (yoga and sports), sun breathing, and being outside in the fresh air.

Nutrition is discussed in detail in the Nutritional Science and Life-Style chapters. As far as treatment with medication is concerned, ayurveda deals exclusively with natural medications derived from plants, animals, and mineral substances. The production of these medications is subject to extremely differentiated principles of pharmacological science. Medication therapy is recommended only after the patient has undergone a cleansing therapy, because it makes little sense to subject a body to medications while it is still filled with toxic substances. Ayurveda first removes the cause of an illness. More often than not, that is the only treatment necessary. This explains why many ayurvedic medications (even when used in extreme doses) do not eliminate the causative agent of an illness when they are tested in a modern laboratory. In a living organism, however, the same substances lead to the elimination of the cause of the illness.

Internal Oil Therapy (*Snehapanam*)

Snehapanam is the internal application of oil substances. This therapy works faster and has more direct effects if the oil is taken undiluted. Not

137

everyone is able to tolerate this. In such cases, the oil is mixed with food. It is very easy to mix the oil with boiled rice. *Snehapanam* has proven very effective for many illnesses, such as hernias and stomach ulcers usually treated surgically.

One day before the scheduled treatment, the patient is put on an anti-*kapha* diet. The last meal is eaten before 6 P.M. The amount of oil given (a minimal, moderate, or maximum dose) has to be determined individually, depending on the age, digestive strength, disturbance of the bio-energy, and the general condition of the patient. The minimal dose is the amount digested within 6 hours; the moderate, within 12 hours; and the maximum dose is the amount digested within 24 hours. To determine a patient's strength of digestion, he is given 1 to 1½ ounces (30–45 ml) of oil on an empty stomach on the first day (after an elimination and a bath). This is followed by drinking 2 ounces (60 ml) of water. The patient then lies down, but does not go to sleep. If the patient is thirsty, he may drink small amounts of water, with or without the addition of ginger powder. It is important to record the time at which the patient believes that the oily substance has been digested. This is determined by when he gets hungry and doesn't taste the oil anymore. He can then eat a light meal, but he should not take a bath.

The result of this procedure determines the dose for the next day's treatment. An attempt is made to increase the dose every day. For instance, if a patient has taken 1 ounce (30 ml) of oil the first day, the dose is increased to 2 ounces (60 ml) the next day. This is repeated for seven days, until the dose is regulated so that on the last day the patient completes digestion within 12 hours. In general, the patient notices an improvement in the digestive process. If the patient needed three hours to digest 1 ounce (30 ml) of the oily substance the first day, the second day he probably will need five hours to digest 2 ounces (60 ml), and eight hours on the third day for 3 ounces (90 ml).

The treatment has been **successful** when *vata* is in balance, the digestion is active, the stool soft and oily, the body soft, and the skin subtle. The treatment has been **excessive** if the patient becomes pale, feels heavy, vomits, feels dizzy, and has undigested food in the stool.

• Indications for using a **minimal dose:** for older people and children who have a weak digestion, and for those who are plagued by chronic fever, diarrhea, and cough, or have little vitality.

• Indications for using a **moderate dose:** boils, blisters, pus, itching, psoriasis, skin disorders, abnormal urine production, rheumatism, and for people who have a moderate digestion and moderate vitality.

- Indications for using a **maximum dose:** gastrointestinal problems, mental illness, trauma, and constipation. High doses can lead to complications, and should be administered only by a physician, and given only to people who are normally able to eat foods that contain large amounts of oil and are able to withstand hunger and thirst.

Rejuvenating and Strengthening Therapy

After pretreatment and cleansing measures have eliminated toxins from the body, and after calming therapy (if necessary), rejuvenating and strengthening therapies can be considered.

One method involves moving the patient into a suitable building. In the early days, these were small houses built far away from everyday commotion. The rooms were totally cut off from the outside world. The only reading materials allowed in these places were philosophical and religious literature. Meditation, prayers, and yoga exercises were highly recommended. After two weeks or longer, the patient would return to the normal world. If possible, these therapies were arranged around the time when *amalaki* fruit was ripe, so that when the person returned to the community, this fruit could be picked directly from the tree.

Another method allows patients to remain in contact with the environment. Yoga exercises, meditation, and prayer are highly recommended to bring the mental processes under control and to refresh the whole person. Further recommendations include walks in a healthy environment, swimming, using music as therapy, and other creative activities.

This therapy's goal is to create a new, positive orientation of personal tendencies and a reorganization of mental, spiritual, and physical habits. During this therapy, it is important to eat easy-to-digest and nutritious foods. The diet should correspond to the patient's bio-type, and should also take the patient's age into consideration.

In addition, several ayurvedic strengthening substances with nutritional value are given to stimulate digestion and to cleanse the channels in the body. These substances serve as tonics. Substances that have particular rejuvenating effects are *Terminalia chebula, Terminalia bellirica, Asparagus racemosus, Hydrocotyle asiatica, Glycyrrhiza glabra, Evolvulus alsinonides, shilajit* (slate oil), detoxified metals, and precious stone oxides from gold, silver, iron, mercury, pearls, diamonds, rubies, and more. *Rasayanas* (rejuvenating substances), such as *amalaki rasayan, aswagandha leha, brahma rasayan, oyavanaprasha, dasamula rasayan, sukumara rasayan,* and *yoga rasayan,* are also used. The latter are more effective when taken on an empty stomach. They should be taken at 12-hour intervals. The dose is one or two teaspoons (15–30 g). In case of a weak digestion, they can be taken with a meal.

139

Index

142